AF334408

Pseudoseizures

Pseudoseizures

Edited by

TERRENCE L. RILEY, M.D.

Associate Professor of Neurology
Boston University Medical Center
Boston, Massachusetts

and

ALEC ROY, M.B., B.Chir. (Cantab)

Associate Professor
Department of Psychiatry
University of Toronto

Staff Psychiatrist
Clarke Institute of Psychiatry
Toronto, Ontario, Canada

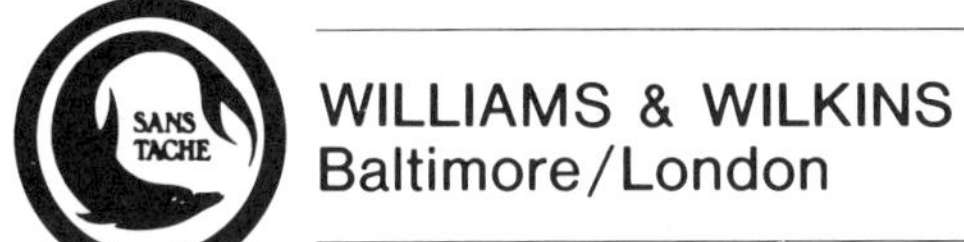

WILLIAMS & WILKINS
Baltimore/London

Copyright ©, 1982
Williams & Wilkins
428 E. Preston Street
Baltimore, Md. 21202, U.S.A.

Made in the United States of America

Library of Congress Cataloging in Publication Data

Main entry under title:

Pseudoseizures.

Includes index.
1. Convulsions. 2. Epilepsy. 3. Hysteria—Complications and sequelae. I. Riley, Terrence L. II. Roy, Alec. [DNLM: 1. Seizures. WL 340 P974]
RC394.C77P76   616.8′45   81-16137
ISBN 0-683-07280-3   AACR2

Composed and printed at the
Waverly Press, Inc.
Mt. Royal and Guilford Aves.
Baltimore, Md. 21202, U.S.A.

For
Ann, Mary, Abigail, and Deirdre
and
Mary and George Roy
and in memory of
Mrs. George Smitten

Foreword

Under a somewhat provocative title, the editors have published a valuable and highly interesting account of the various periodic syndromes met with in neuropsychiatric practice.

The lush symptomatology of epilepsy naturally occupies the foreground and prompts one to pose two basic questions. To start with, how does one define epilepsy? Secondly, what are the pathognomonic features of a genuine epileptic attack?

Let us take these two fundamental questions in turn. Hughlings Jackson spoke of "a sudden excessive discharge of gray matter," but this is an attempt to explain rather than to define. Clinically, the most conspicuous manifestation is the appearance at intervals of a disturbance of consciousness, or perhaps it would be better to say awareness. Sometimes the recurring episode entails spontaneous, unwilled and uncontrollable movement, ranging in degree from a twitch to a convulsion. These two prime features do not necessarily coexist; obtundity may not entail motor phenomena, and vice versa. Indeed one contributor gives a detailed account of some oddities of neurological practice characterized by periodic spells of ungovernable motility (paroxysmal choreoathetosis, porphyria, cataplexy). But these events do not easily fit into the cadre of epilepsy. Again, the presenting feature may comprise remitting disturbed behavior as in the various unprovoked, aggressive or explosive states. Finally one has to decide whether any intrinsic anomaly of cerebral function underlies the periodic attributes of epilepsy whatever their nature. Here then would be an important distinction between epilepsy and some other cyclical disorders like migraine or periodic paralysis. The suspicion of an epileptic *Grundstörung* cannot therefore be dismissed out of hand. One could readily imagine a *morbus comitialis sine epilepsia.*

This idea deserves consideration. Does epilepsy imply something besides the obvious intermittent and clinically dramatic episodes? Kinnier Wilson used to tell of a patient of his who had her first fit on the day of her menarche. Her second and presumably last seizure occurred at the end of her menopause. "How should we categorize such a case?" he asked.

No one with neurological experience would make light of the difficulties that may bedevil the confident diagnosis of epilepsy. Some consultants practice for years without ever witnessing a fit. Rarely has the physician had the chance of viewing the incident which precipitated a particular medical interview. The patient may have been alone at the time. Or, an untrained bystander, taken by surprise, can supply no observations of real importance. Maybe neither the patient nor his family is English-speaking.

The advent of electroencephalography has not altogether resolved the clinician's doubts and difficulties. There are times when they have even been enhanced. Likewise the frequent abuse of powerful anticonvulsants can raise questions that confuse rather than clarify.

Years ago, Féré said that there are as many epilepsies as there are epileptics. Once again we witness what applies throughout Medicine, namely the realization that no two patients are identical. Kinnier Wilson—whom we recall chiefly because of his interest in basal ganglionic disorders—was in his day even more an epileptologist. He never ceased to ordain that one should always speak of "the epilepsies," for he was sceptical of any such entity as Maisonneuve's "idiopathic" epilepsy.

Naturally the syncopes come up for earnest consideration and they are ably described by Dr. Riley in his important chapter. Obviously the subject is anything but simple. Syncopal attacks associated with convulsive manifestations are not to be overlooked. In the same way, the hyperventilation syndromes only too often muddy the waters of differential diagnosis.

Dr. Riley quotes the intriguing study made by Gastaut and Gastaut (1968) into the ultimate explanation which emerged after an intensive study of 946 patients referred to them because of episodic attacks of unconsciousness. Epilepsy was found to be the explanation in 377 subjects and syncope in 417 instances.

When considering a putative case of epilepsy, Bender's "transient global amnesia" (TGA) must not be overlooked. In some of the reported cases the electroencephalographic findings were suspicious. On balance, however, disorders of the cerebral vasculature appear to be more probable than does a latent epilepsy. Also of diagnostic importance is Guilleminault's fascinating "neutral state syndrome." This not very appropriate title comprises somnosis interspersed with spells of semi-automatic behavior, of which there is no subsequent recollection.

Alcoholic blackouts are episodes of amnesia rather than of unconsciousness, but they are important in forensic diagnosis. Kraepelin's "poriomania" or "la maladie du juif errant" is yet another condition which may lead to medicolegal repercussions. Strictly speaking, poriomania refers to relatively long-lasting ambulatory fugue states typically preceded by a convulsive seizure. Often a vivid psychiatric coloring pervades the picture. Recovery is usually abrupt and the subject cannot recall where he has been or what he has done, though his behavior may not necessarily have been inappropriate during this interlude. Stengel's diagnostic triad makes seductive reading in this connection but is not wholly convincing.

These considerations lead naturally to the clinical phenomenon which Charcot called "hystero-epilepsy." This expression has not been universally adopted, and we are encouraged to refer to them as psychogenic seizures. Simulated epilepsy is a thing apart, an instance of play-acting or deliberate aberrant behavior rather than of subconscious psychopathology.

The contributors emphasize the all-important point that psychogenic pseudoseizures often complicate the clinical course of a known chronic epileptic and may lead to considerable difficulties in management, drug treatment and prognosis. Dr. Fenton's term "pseudoepileptic seizure" is preferred to Charcot's nomenclature. Attention is directed to the hazards of misdiagnosis at the time of the original interview, with its probable instigation of inappropriate medication. Seventeen patients diagnosed as epileptics and treated for years with anticonvulsants turned out to have had all along nothing but hysterical attacks. One patient had been elected Chairman of the local Epileptic Society. Another had become Secretary of a local Society. Yet, neither rightly fitted into the category of the chronic epileptic.

The incidence of feigned epilepsy must surely be rare, except in a few very special and unusual circumstances. Some of our senior neurologists will remember the wartime and immediate postwar "schools" where "doctors" deliberately taught the technique of evading military service by feigning epileptic seizures and by producing bogus medical certificates and faked prescriptions.

This leads to the second of the two basic questions mentioned earlier, namely just what are the signs which may be accepted as pathognomonic of an epileptic attack. The usual criteria, namely tongue-biting, self-injury, and incontinence, are, it must be admitted, very occasionally present in pseudoseizures or in syncope. Perhaps the most reliable hallmark of a true epileptic attack is a Babinski response. Hammond's case has been quoted as evidence to the contrary, but that particular instance was self-induced. Anyone who can deliberately mimic a seizure has no doubt also been taught the trick of cocking-up the great toe at the appropriate moment.

Perhaps, too, Dr. Trimble's raised prolactin level may turn out to be an invaluable indication of whether a particular incident is or is not truly epileptic.

The last two chapters are of compelling interest and in some respects form the most important section of this volume. Medicolegal issues are constantly arising irrespective of whether the accusation involves a victim of pseudoepilepsy or epilepsy. It is difficult for a medical expert witness to impress the logical thinking of the judicature. Dr. Rodin ruefully quotes the outcome of the Detroit Psychosurgery Trial but one's personal approval is with a court which ruled that prisoners or inmates of state institutions cannot in any circumstances give voluntary consent to medical research into the causes of their behavior, especially if it involves depth electrography.

Chapter 13 deals with the legal aspects of pseudoseizures. It is a most valuable contribution. Perhaps the problem of responsibility is best summed up in the author's concluding words, to the effect that the outcome may turn on "the skill of the respective advocates."

Macdonald Critchley
Old Sodbury, Avon

Preface

One of the editors of this volume is a Neurologist and the other a Psychiatrist. Both developed an interest in this subject as a direct consequence of clinical contact with patients with pseudoseizures. One of us (TLR) also made an informal survey of 30 university departments of neurology. It was estimated that approximately 5% of all admissions for uncontrollable seizures were for patients eventually found not to have epilepsy at all, while approximately 10% of admissions were for patients with epilepsy whose current seizures were thought to be mainly pseudoseizures.

Among outpatients, the survey respondents estimated that approximately 10–20% of their seizure patients had either pseudoseizures alone or in addition to epileptic seizures.

Thus, the idea for this volume came from both the realization that this was not an uncommon clinical problem and the appreciation of the difficulties in diagnosis and management that these patients can present. We were unaware of any volume that dealt specifically with these issues. We felt there was a need for such a book and hope this volume will prove interesting and useful.

Terrence L. Riley, M.D.
Alec Roy, M.B., B.Chir.(Cantab)

Contributors

Michael P. Alexander, M.D., Chief, Aphasia Unit, Boston Veterans Administration Medical Center, Associate Professor, Department of Neurology, Boston University School of Medicine, Boston, MA

Jacqueline Cummins-Ducharme, M.S.W., Clinical Instructor of Neurology Boston University School of Medicine, Boston, MA

Robert G. Feldman, M.D., Professor and Chairman, Department of Neurology, Professor of Pharmacology, Boston University School of Medicine, Chief, Neurology Services, University Hospital and Boston Veterans Administration Medical Center, Boston, MA

Thomas G. Gutheil, M.D., Director, Program in Psychiatry and the Law at Massachusetts Mental Health Center, Associate Professor of Psychiatry, Harvard Medical School, Visiting Lecturer, Harvard Law School, President, Law and Psychiatry Resource Center, Boston, MA

E. Wayne Massey, M.D., Assistant Professor of Neurology, Duke University Medical Center, Durham, N.C.

Mark J. Mills, J.D., M.D., Commissioner, Department of Mental Health, Boston, MA

David I. Mostofsky, Ph.D., Professor of Psychology, Boston University, Boston, MA

J. D. Parkes, F.R.C.P., D.P.M., Senior Lecturer, University Department of Neurology, King's College Hospital and the Institute of Psychiatry, Honorary Consultant Neurologist, King's College Hospital and The Maudsley Hospital, Denmark Hill, London

Norman L. Paul, M.D., Clinical Associate Professor, Department of Neurology, Boston University School of Medicine, Boston, MA

Terrence L. Riley, M.D., Associate Professor, Department of Neurology, Boston University School of Medicine, Director, EEG and Sleep Laboratories, University Hospital, Boston, MA

Ernst A. Rodin, M.D., Medical Director, Epilepsy Center of Michigan, Director, Division of Clinical Neurophysiology, Department of Neurology, Henry Ford Hospital, Detroit, MI, Clinical Professor of Neurology, University of Michigan, Ann Arbor, MI

Alec Roy, M.B., B.Chir. (Cantab), D.P.M. M.Phil., M.R.C.P., M.R.C. Psych., F.R.C.P.(C.), Associate Professor, Department of Psychiatry, University of Toronto, Staff Psychiatrist, Clarke Institute of Psychiatry, Toronto, Ontario, Canada

Donald F. Scott, F.R.C.P., D.P.M., Consultant in Charge EEG Department, Section of Neurological Sciences, London Hospital, Whitechapel, London

Michael Trimble, M.B., BSc, M. Phil., M.R.C.P., M.R.C. Psych., Consultant Physician in Psychological Medicine, National Hospital for Nervous Diseases, Queen Square, London

Daniel T. Williams, M.D., Assistant Professor of Clinical Psychiatry, Columbia College of Physicians and Surgeons, Director, Pediatric Neuropsychiatry Service, Columbia-Presbyterian Medical Center, New York, NY

Contents

PSYCHIATRIC ASPECTS

Chapter 1 The History of Epilepsy and Hysteria

E. WAYNE MASSEY, M.D.

ANCIENT TIMES

Among the primitive Homoric Greeks (pre-Hippocratic) concepts of brain function and behavior were based on a religion of fear. The Olympian or celestial gods were believed to inflict or avert disease at will, particularly epidemic diseases. For example, the chthonia were infernal gods who caused epilepsy, insanity and hysteria (Temkin, 1936, 1945). Epilepsy was assumed by ancient Greeks to be a miasma cast upon us by the "plots of Hecate and the invasions of Heros."

Hysterical symptoms were recorded in the Egyptian Papyri 4000 years ago, but the word itself first appeared in writings attributed to Hippocrates and reflected the belief that the womb floated about in the body causing symptoms wherever it came to rest.

Hippocratic contributions to neurology include his tract on "The Sacred Disease" written in 400 BC as an attempt to comment on the superstition associated with epilepsy (Hippocrates, trans. 1932).

> They who first referred this disease (epilepsy) to the gods appear to me to have been just such persons as the conjurers, pureficators, mountebanks, and charlatans now are, who give themselves out as being excessively religious and as knowing more than other people ... Neither, in truth, do I count it a worthy opinion to hold that the body of man is polluted by God, the most impure by the most holy; for were it defiled or did it suffer from any other thing, it would likely be purified and sanctified rather than polluted by God .... But this disease seems to me to be no wise more divine than others; but it has its nature such as other diseases have, and a cause whence it originates and its nature and cause are divine only just as much as all others, unless when from length of time it is confirmed and has

> become stronger than the remedies applied. Its origin is hereditary like that of other diseases.

Hippocrates also gave clinical descriptions of seizures which were unique in their quality at that time. He noted that seizures may be hereditary and that they were accompanied by incontinences and foaming of saliva around the mouth. He described unilateral seizures as well as the aura preceding seizures, "but such persons as are inhabited by the disease know beforehand when they are about to be seized and flee from men either to their homes or to a deserted place and cover themselves up. This they do from shame of the affliction and not from the fear of divinity as many suppose." Hippocrates believed that the site of the disorder in epilepsy was in the brain, which to him was the organ of the senses—emotion and intellect (Garrison, 1929). His writings contain antiquity's best discussion of the brain (Penfield, 1958). It is a magnificent statement that could have been written only by a physician who had studied epileptic patients and their seizures.

In *Epidemics* Hippocrates describes "puerperal hemiplegia" and convulsions with a paralysis of the right arm and loss of speech.

> A woman who lived on the sea front was seized with a fever while in the third month of pregnancy. She was immediately seized with pains in the loins. On the third day she had pain in the head, neck and around about the right clavicle. Very shortly the tongue became unable to articulate and the right arm was paralyzed following a convulsion as happens in hemiplegia. Her speech was delirious; speech was indistinct but she was no longer paralyzed. About the fourteenth day she reached a crisis and the fever left her (Temkin, 1933).

Greek medicine was established in Rome by Asclepiades of Bithynia (circa 124 BC) who described the "frenzy" occurring in epilepsy and separated it from symptoms of drug abuse common at that time. Aurelius Cornelius Celsus (25 BC to 50 AD), a physician to emperors Tiberius and Caligula, described the treatment of epilepsy in his *De Re Medicina* (Temkin, 1947). He noted the difficulty in curing epilepsy after it had become established at a certain age. Epilepsy was called "morbus comitialis." Its treatment was detailed, even to the extent of prescribing sexual intercourse (incorporating warm blood of slain gladiators) for boys with an obstinate case of epilepsy. Soranus of Ephesus (McHenry, 1969) and Aretaeus of Cappadocia (Ilberg, 1923) also contributed descriptions of epilepsy.

Hysteroepilepsy is reported in the Bible in Numbers 24:4 and I Samuel 19:24 and resuscitation of a cataleptic or hysteroepileptic child is mentioned in I Kings (18:17–23) and also in Matthew (9:18, 23–25). In the

Talmud, epilepsy is attributed to coitus under bizarre conditions. Its hereditary nature is recognized since marriage into epileptic families is interdicted (Brim, 1943).

Galen of Pergamus added anatomical findings and physiological concepts relating to nervous diseases including epilepsy (Galen, 1934; Fulton, 1956; Major, 1961). Caelius Aurelianus had notions of differences between convulsive and comatose forms of epilepsy and the tendency of victims of vertigo to become epileptic (Drabkin, 1950). Ancient writers in general believed that epilepsy was due to an accumulation of pituitous humors in the cerebral ventricles and that the symptoms were the efforts of nature to relieve pressure. Galen had placed the origin of epilepsy in the brain but believed that it might also proceed from the stomach or from most distant organs indicated by the aura which marked its onset.

MIDDLE AGES

Epilepsy in the Middle Ages and Renaissance was regarded as a contagious disease, as in the chthonian cult of the ancient Greeks, and an isolation hospital for epileptics was founded at the Cloister of St. Valentine at Rufach (Upper Alsace) in 1486. Significant rational contributions to the clinical phenomena of epilepsy were nevertheless made by Bernard of Gordon (Lennox, 1941), teacher in Montpellier from 1285–1307:

> Epilepsy is a disease of the brain, removing sensation, motion, and erection from the whole body, accompanied by a very serious disturbance of movement, because of an occlusion made in the non-principle ventricles of the brain . . . . If the principle ventricles of the brain were to be occluded, it would be apoplexy . . . in apoplexy the great and principle ventricles are occluded, but in epilepsy the small ones . . . . The paroxysm of epilepsy is short, and not of itself fatal, but a paroxysm of apoplexy is continuous 'till death, which comes in a short time. If it happens that the paroxysm passes off in four days, the patient will be freed, but will lapse into paralysis.

Arnold of Villanova (Storch and Storch, 1939) and John of Gaddesden (Lennox, 1939), a physician to Edward II of England, also contributed to the knowledge of epilepsy, with reports of cases and religious interpretations of origins.

SEVENTEENTH AND EIGHTEENTH CENTURY

In the seventeenth century, William Harvey brought together the concepts of his predecessors on functions of the nervous system by using anatomical research. His contributions to clinical neurology included descriptions of epileptic seizures (Brain, 1959; Hunter and McAlpine, 1957), noting some presumably focal features.

Electrophysiology had its origin with Luigi Galvani (Fulton and Cushing, 1936), who studied electrical phenomena in animals. Subsequently, Alden Galvani performed electrical stimulation in human bodies following decapitation. William Heberden, the great London practitioner, wrote on many subjects including epilepsy (Heberden, 1802), expanding somewhat on clinical observations. Tissot also studied epilepsy and described many of the hospital cases he saw during that period (Tissot, 1770; Bucher, 1958). John Cooke, at the London Hospital, wrote a section about epilepsy from his work with the Croonian lectures (Cooke, 1820–1823). Although these various clinical reports mentioned some associated diseases, there were few insightful explanations of epilepsy or interictal behavior from reporters of this era.

NINETEENTH CENTURY

As time progressed, despite more knowledge of the function of the brain, little was added to man's notion of epilepsy. Fear and superstitions associated with disease persisted, and the concept of epilepsy as a specific neurological entity amenable to treatment did not develop until the nineteenth century. At the turn of the century, William Heberden, in his *Commentaries*, showed that although the pathology of epilepsy was poorly understood, the general clinical treatment of the disease could be performed on a rational basis (Heberden, 1802). He emphasized that the frequency of seizures was variable and that in some patients several fits might occur in a day, while in other patients seizures may be dormant for many years. Children were more likely to have fits but to recover from attacks more easily than adults. Male cases seemed to predominate and the condition appeared to be partially hereditary. Heberden suggested that physicians not confuse epilepsy with the usual childhood convulsions and that during epileptic convulsion the patient was not to be manipulated—all treatment being administered only before or after the ictus.

Scientific study of epilepsy was implemented by the separation of epileptic patients from the insane and mental hospitals by Esquirol and Pinel and was part of the general movement toward the more humane treatment of the mentally ill. Most of the classical studies of epilepsy which appeared in France and England in the nineteenth century derived from the work of physicians such as Charcot and Gowers who were associated with asylums for the insane, special hospitals for epileptics, or the epileptic wards of general hospitals.

The subsequent terminology or separation of specific types of epilepsy developed gradually in the nineteenth century. Esquirol, a psychiatrist at the Salpêtrière, wrote that attacks alternate in intensity, and there were both severe and slight attacks, which he called "le grand mal" and "le petit mal" (1883). Although "grand mal" meant a generalized convulsion, the meaning of "petit mal" remained vague. Another early French psychiatrist, Louis Florentine Calmeil, in his thesis on epilepsy introduced the term "absence" characterized by passing mental confusion (Calmeil, 1824). The lack of clarity of Galen's use of the word "aura" was remedied by Prichard (1882) and later by Rhomberg (1853) who stated that premonitory symptoms may be of a "sensitive, motor or physical character."

Jules Germain Francois Maisonneuve (1804) initiated the traditional division of epilepsy into idiopathic and symptomatic classes. He considered that the idiopathic type was due to congenital, spontaneous, plethoric or humoral causes and that the symptomatic was due to "irritation" of the brain. Portal, in a classic treatise on epilepsy (1827) after years of clinical observation and postmortem studies, believed the seat of epilepsy was always in the brain, particularly in its medullary part, and from there electrically or humorally propagated via the nerves to the various parts of the body.

To understand the early nineteenth century concept of epilepsy, it is necessary to review the basic rules of early physiologists concerning nervous system function. Flourens believed that irritability and sensibility were assigned to different parts of the nervous system (1823). The cerebral hemisphere and cerebellum, however, were not irritable, because it appeared that movements could not be elicited by stimulation of the cerebral hemisphere, i.e., by Flourens' methods of electrical stimulation. Irritability pertained only to the spinal cord, its continuation in the medulla oblongata, and its end in the corpora quadrigemina (midbrain). These parts alone, particulary the medulla oblongata, had the property of exciting muscular contraction. The cerebral hemispheres were the seat of volition and sensation but not movement. On the basis of this concept of nervous function, Hall (1851, 1852) decided the medulla was the site of origin of convulsions. Loss of consciousness was thought to be due either to excessive vascular engorgement of the brain or the opposite, anemia of the brain. A similar view was held by Copeland (1850).

From his research with Claude Bernard on vasomotor phenomena, Brown-Séquard (1856, 1860) postulated that excitation of the spinal cord or the base of the brain caused reflex sympathetic vasoconstriction to the face as well as to the brain to produce anemia. He noted that "the brain proper loses at once its function just as it does in complete syncope." He did not agree that the spinal cord itself was the origin of epilepsy. In his studies of the transverse sections of the spinal cord he could produce convulsions, particularly if the skin were pinched:

> Even in cases of epilepsy due to a disease of the encephalon, the cause of the fits may originate from some points of the skin, and the prevention of the passage of the aura, in such cases, can prevent the fits. There are four cases of this kind that I know, in three of which the disease consisted in a tumor in the brain. In my animals the same thing exists; although the alteration of the spinal cord—which is the cause of epilepsy so far as I have been able to ascertain, ceases. The aura may originate from any part of any centripetal nerve, and there is no doubt that its place varies according to the location of disease in the nervous centres, when it is due to such a disease.

Although he described the manner in which these convulsions resembled epileptic seizures, Brown-Séquard felt that they had different origin from true epileptic seizures. He suggested that epilepsy was a reflex phenomenon.

Histological examination of the brain allowed postulation of more precise sites of origin of epilepsy. Schroeder van der Kolk (1859), well acquainted with Brown-Séquard's experimental studies of the medulla oblongata, was impressed that it was the center of many reflex functions. He regarded "an exalted sensibility and excitability" of the ganglion centers of the medulla oblongata as the first cause of epilepsy. From these convulsions arose an involuntary reflex movement causing disturbance of circulation of the vasomotor nerves.

In Bright's anatomical studies, lesions of the cerebral cortex had been found in certain cases of epilepsy (1836). He reported cases of unilateral seizures, noting their connection with impaired vision, paresthesia and weakness of the convulsed part and with preservation of consciousness. His belief, based on Foville's views on the functional preponderance of gray matter in the brain, was that the site of origin of epilepsy was lesions affecting the membrane or cortex of the opposite surface of the brain. Robert Bently Todd, physician to Kings College Hospital, was familiar with all types of epilepsy and interested in seizures appearing in the course of uremia or as a consequence of poisoning (McIntyre, 1956). He proposed a humoral theory of epilepsy and noted that an epileptic attack left the brain in an exhausted condition which may lead to a hemiplegic paralysis (Todd's paralysis) (1855).

Jean Martin Charcot (1825–1893), the greatest neurologist of France, Professor of Pathology and later of Neurology on the Faculty of Medicine at the Salpêtriere, contributed significantly to understanding of epilepsy and its distinction from hysteria (Beeson, 1928; Garrison, 1925).

On his wards he had some women with "convulsions" who were
epileptics and others who were hysterics who had learned to imitate
epileptic attacks. Charcot strove to discover means of distinguishing
hysterical and epileptic convulsions. These "hystero-epileptics" often
included such diverse groups as epileptic old women who preferred to
endure the seizures rather than to take bromides and hysterical girls
who had been abandoned to the hospital by relatives. Many of the
hysterical young women, who became rather attached to Charcot,
through constant association with the epileptics began to mimic convulsions of major epilepsy. Charcot developed a complex classification
of hysteria and epilepsy.

The hysterical seizure usually contained elaborate and spectacular
features:

> The patient loses consciousness and the paroxysm proper begins. It is
> divided into four periods which are quite clear and distinct. In the first, the
> patient executes certain epileptiform convulsive movements. Then comes
> the period of great gesticulations of salutation, which are of extreme
> violence, interrupted from time to time by an arching of the body which is
> absolutely characteristic; the trunk being bent bow fashion sometimes in
> front (emprosthotonos), sometimes backwards (opisthotonos), the feet and
> head alone touching the bed, the body constituting the arch. During this
> time the patient utters wild cries. Then comes the third period, called the
> period of passional attitudes during which he utters words and cries in
> relation with the sad delirium and terrifying visions which pursue
> him . . . . Finally, he regains consciousness, recognizes the persons around
> him and calls them by name, but the delirium and hallucinations continue
> for some time . . . . Never during the course of these cries has he bitten his
> tongue or wet his bed (Havens, 1966) (Fig. 1.1).

According to Freud, Charcot was the first to demonstrate that hysterical manifestations could be removed or reproduced by hypnosis,
and Freud concluded that this proved a psychological origin (Freud,
1959).

However, not all his colleagues admired his work, as Axel Munthe
wrote in *The Story of San Michele* (1930):

> I seldom failed to attend Professor Charcot's famous Lecons due Mardi
> in the Salpêtrière, just then chiefly devoted to his grande hysterie and to
> hypnotism. The huge amphitheatre was filled to the last place with a
> multicolored audience drawn from tout Paris . . . full of morbid curiosity to
> witness the startling phenomena of hypnotism almost forgotten since the
> days of Mesmer and Braid . . . . Some of these subjects were no doubt real
> somnambulists faithfully carrying out in a waking state the various sugges-
> tions made to them during sleep—post-hypnotic suggestions. Many of them

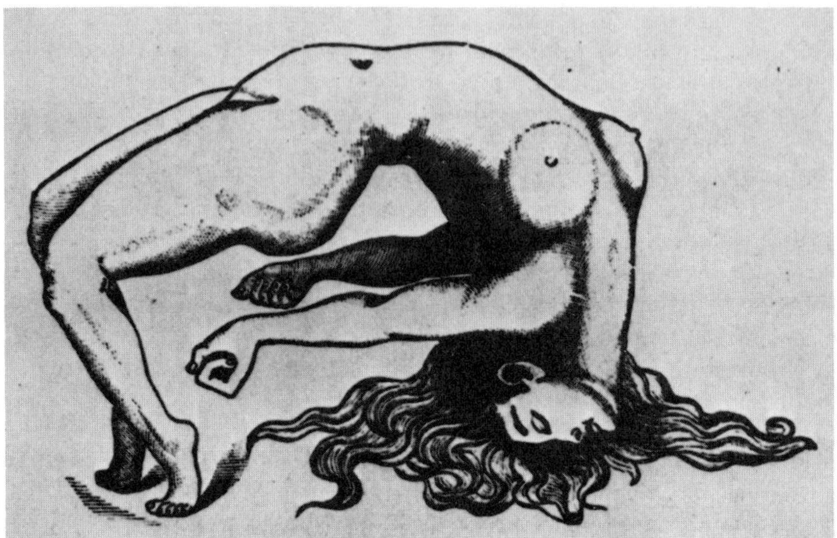

Figure 1.1.   Drawing of patient with hysteroepilepsy demonstrates "Arc de Cercle" of Gilles de la Tourette. (Courtesy of L. McHenry, M.D., In *Garrison's History of Neurology*, 1969.).

were mere frauds, knowing quite well what they were expected to do, delighted to perform their various tricks in public, cheating of the hysterics. They were always read to 'piquer une attaque' of Charcot's classical grande hystérie, arc-en-ciel and all, or to exhibit his famous three states of hypnotism: lethargy, catalepsy, somnambulism, all invented by the Master and hardly ever observed outside the Salpêtrière. Some of them smelt with delight a bottle of ammonia when told it was rose water, others would eat a piece of charcoal when presented to them as chocolate. Another would crawl on all fours on the floor, barking furiously, when told she was a dog, flap her arms as if trying to fly when a glove was thrown at her feet with a suggestion of being a snake. Another would walk with a top hat in her arms rocking it to and fro and kissing it tenderly when she was told it was her baby. Hypnotized right and left, dozens of times a day, by doctors and many of these unfortunate girls spent their days in a state of semitrance; their brains bewildered by all sorts of absurd suggestions, half conscious and certainly not responsible for their doings, sooner or later doomed to end their days in the salles des agites if not in a lunatic asylum.

In Russia, the first professor of nervous and mental diseases at Moscow, Aleksea Yahovlevich Kozhevnikov, made the original elaboration of epilepsy partialis continuans (1895).

John Hughlings Jackson, father of English neurology, was appointed as physician to the National Hospital in 1862 (Critchley, 1960). His more than 300 papers include meticulous observations of the clinical, pathological and physiological aspects of neurological diseases. He is remembered primarily for his three contributions to the fundamental principles of neurological thought or theory—namely, on epilepsy, on aphasia and on the doctrine of levels of function of the nervous system.

Focal seizures, motor, sensory and those with physical disturbance, occupied Jackson's attention. His studies on epilepsy, "sudden excessive temporary discharge of nervous tissue," primarily concern convulsions beginning unilaterally (1861, 1863). He demonstrated that a seizure may begin in the thumb, face or the great toe and spread up the limb in a constant manner. "Such unilateral seizures may become generalized, but usually begin in those cortical areas that have the largest representation." Jackson also noted that the distribution and order of involvement of this part is the same in unilateral seizures as in a hemiplegia. From these clinical observations he developed a concept of localization of function within the cortex that was later confirmed by the experimental observations of Hitzig and Ferrier (Broadbent, 1903; Greenblatt, 1965). Hughlings Jackson's concept of the development of unilateral seizures was a cornerstone in the study of epilepsy (Walshe, 1961; Riese, 1956). It is of note that he seemed to believe that many of the alleged "hysterical" spells had an origin common to epileptic seizures.

His contemporary, Gowers, described a clinical picture of all types of seizures and disturbances of awareness. He differentiated idiopathic from organic epilepsy, pointing out that a lesion at or near the motor regions of the cerebral cortex caused seizures (1881, 1909). His concept of epilepsy was based on the theory of an imbalance in the continuous flow of nervous energy. He believed that in epilepsy the equilibrium or natural balance was fragile; a sudden escape of energy from the normal control should result in a spontaneous discharge, or seizure. He realized that a single convulsion, however characteristic, did not constitute epilepsy, the condition of chronically unstable control of nervous energy.

Gowers did much to separate epilepsy from hysteria. The "hysterical," "hysteroid," "hysteroepileptic" or "hysteria major" attack had spasmodic movements of a more or less coordinated character and, since the muscular contraction was produced at will, the spasm had a rather purposive aspect (Gowers, 1885). He emphasized that the "rigid fixation of the trunk and limbs alternates with wild movements in which the limbs are thrown about; the arms strike out, the legs kick, the head is dashed side to side. These phenomena are interrupted by periods of comparative tranquility."

The attacks could be without warning and vary in severity and character. Consciousness was "changed" rather than "lost." Emphasizing the requirement for use of restraints in some individuals, he noted friends of the patient might observe "six persons had to sit on him to keep him down."

Gowers repeated the differentiating points of Charcot and Richern in hysterical seizures:

1. The attack is often preceded by a peculiar mental state, with hallucinations, and is frequently accompanied by transient contractures of one or another limb.
2. The tonic spasm with which the epileptoid state commences is usually immediately preceded by violent movements of the limbs.
3. An attack may be brought on by compressing the ovaries or in some cases by touching certain "hysterogenic points."
4. At any period of the attack it may be instantly arrested by ovarian compression.
5. These attacks were not influenced by appropriate epilepsy treatment but by that suitable for hysteria.

Gowers emphasized that the "ovarian compression," a crucial test of Charcot, was rarely successful in England and unknowningly predicted cultural influence upon features of psychological disease.

S. Weir Mitchell (1829–1914), the father of American neurology, is known for his monumental study of peripheral nerve injuries (1872). However, his fame during his own lifetime was based primarily on the rest treatment which he used in cases of hysteria, including hystero-epilepsy (1875).

ELECTROENCEPHALOGRAM

Hans Berger, Professor of Psychiatry and later Rector of the University of Jeha, first succeeded in recording the electrical activity of the brain through the intact skull by adding a vacuum tube as an amplifier to a string galvanometer, after the improvements of Einthoven allowed further studies of the exposed cortex (Ginzberg, 1949; Haymaker, 1953). Richard Canton, Professor of Physiology at Liverpool, first discovered electrical potentials from the exposed cortical surface of the rabbit brain (Brazier, 1955). In 1929, Berger studied and named the electroencephalogram, finding two major rhythms: alpha and beta (in normals). He also demonstrated that wave characteristics could be used as an index of brain disease. Berger's work, published in a series of 19 papers from 1929–1938, was ridiculed. But in 1937 he was invited to preside with Adrian at a Paris symposium on the electrical activity of the brain. After Edgar Douglas (Lord) Adrian verified the nature of the Berger rhythm, Berger's efforts were recognized (1934). Adrian also performed other classical work in physiology and shared the Nobel Prize in Physiology and Medicine in 1932.

The first description of epileptic patterns in the electroencephlogram was made in 1912 in experimental seizures in animals (Brazier, 1960). Berger, however, first recorded and described an electroencephalogram of an epileptic patient. The classical studies of different epileptic electroencephalographic patterns, including the 3 cps spike and wave in petit mal, were described by Gibbs (1935) and H.H. Jasper and L. Carmichal (1935). Gray Walter (1936) first recognized that brain tumors can be located through the skull by abnormal slow waves in the surrounding tissue.

TREATMENT OF EPILEPSY

Each era in the history of the treatment of epilepsy had its own concept and each physician had his own drugs. Zinc oxide, silver preparations, turpentine, indigo, belladonna and inhalation of chloroform were among the greatest remedies. The first breakthrough in the treatment of epilepsy came in May 1857, when Sir Charles Locock (1799–1875) discussed a paper on epilepsy read before the Royal Medical and Chirurgical Society of London by Sir Edward H. Sieveking. He reported that bromides had been used successfully in the treatment of hysterical epilepsy (Lennox, 1957). Sieveking, one of the early physicians in the National Hospital, had made a thorough study of all aspects of epilepsy. With the beneficial results of treatment with bromides that followed, Sir Samuel Wilkes (1859, 1866) urged their general use in the treatment of epilepsy. Hughlings Jackson (1861) commented on the use of bromides as originally suggested by Wilkes. Gowers used bromides but tried other drugs also. The next significant step came with the introduction of the barbituric acid derivatives by Alfred Hauptmann (1912). The discovery of the effectiveness of diphenylhydantoin by Merritt and Putman in 1938 was one of the major landmarks in the history of modern neurology (1938, 1939).

MASS HYSTERIA

Epidemics of various movement disorders began in the Middle Ages, with the description of dancing mania often associated with infectious epidemics or occurring in forms of group hysteria. Epidemics of epilepsy, a form of mass hysteria, were not unknown during the seventeenth and eighteenth century (Fig. 1.2). Religious houses particularly appear to have been subject to these disturbances. Richer in *Etudes Cliniques sur la Grande Hysterie* (1885) described a number of epidemics and Aldous Huxley in *The Devils of London* (1957) vividly portrays a

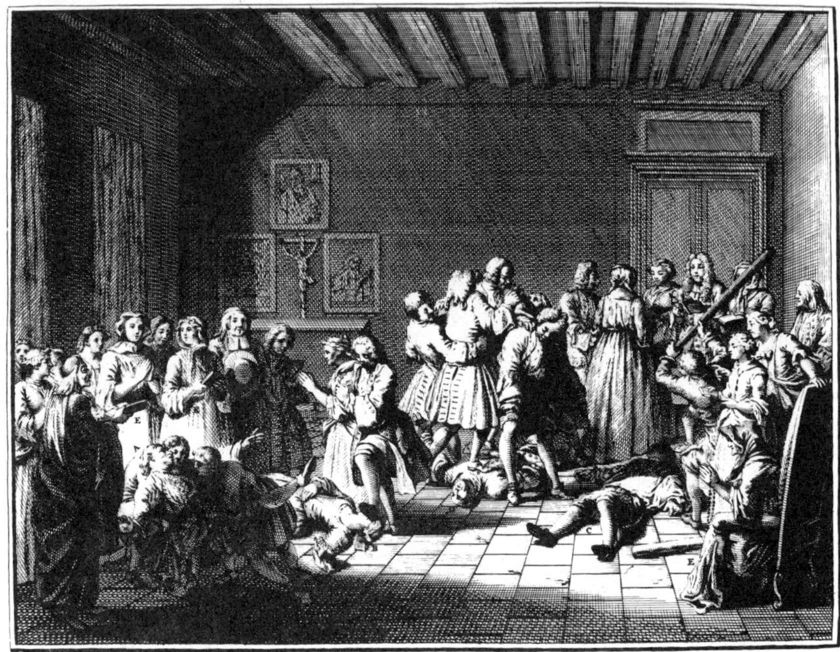

Figure 1.2. "Agitations des Convulsionaires" shows an epidemic of convulsions, a form of mass hysteria, not uncommon in seventeenth and eighteenth century. (Courtesy of The Wellcome Trustees, London.)

famous disturbance in an Ursuline convent. To illustrate the frequency of hysterical epilepsy in the nineteenth century, one need only review the experience of Charcot's special ward at the Salpêtrière.

Epidemics, of course, are not unique to Western culture: amok, a sudden outburst of wild rage among Malaysian natives; latah, the startled reaction seen in Malaysian people; piblokta or "Arctic hysteria" when the patient begins to scream, tear off his clothing and throw himself in the snow or ice, as seen among the Eskimoes. Voodoo, practiced in African societies, reveals an increased incidence between hysterical and epileptic disorders. Among the American religious movements the occurrence of the "jerks" perhaps would be an example of group hysteria. Outbreaks of psychosomatic illness in rural elementary schools have been reported, usually in the form of hyperventilation. Over 100 reports were published in the nineteenth century but far less reports of epidemic hysteria have been reported in the United States.

EPILEPSY AND HYSTERIA IN LITERATURE

Epilepsy has been included in literary writing throughout the centuries but space allows mention of only a few.

The Bible

With the introduction in the New English Bible of the word "convulsions" for "straight away the spirit tare him" and "goes rigid" for the words "pineth away," the story of the boy at the foot of the Mount of Transfiguration reads in parts like a modern case history:

> A man in the crowd spoke up: "Master, I brought my son to you. He is possessed by a spirit which makes him speechless. Whenever it attacks him, it dashes him to the ground and he foams at the mouth, grinds his teeth, and goes rigid. I asked your disciples to cast it out, but they failed." Jesus answered: "What an unbelieving and perverse generation! How long shall I be with you? How long must I endure you? Bring him to me." So they brought the boy to him; and as soon as the spirit saw him it threw the boy into convulsions, and he fell on the ground and rolled about foaming at the mouth. Jesus asked his father, "How long has it been like this?" "From childhood," he replied, "often it has tried to make an end of him by throwing him into the fire or into water ...." Jesus rebuked the unclean spirit. "Deaf and dumb spirit," he said, "I command you, come out of him and never go back!" After crying aloud and racking him fiercely, it came out, and the boy looked like a corpse; in fact, many said, "He is dead." But Jesus took his hand and raised him to his feet, and he stood up (Mark 9:17–27).

This is a remarkable description of a grand mal seizure, likely idiopathic epilepsy. The assumption that the illness was due to possession by the spirit (madness was supposed to be due to demon possession) was common.

In Luke 9:39–42, in a parallel version, a cry, "he suddenly crieth out," or "sudden scream" precedes the convulsions and the evil spirit is stated to be the devil in the latter part of the passage. In Matthew 17:15–18, the same narrative is also abbreviated and the word "lunatick" becomes "epileptic" in the New English Bible.* The father says: "Have pity, sir, on my son; he is an epileptic and has bad fits, and he keeps falling about, often into the fire, often into water."

A man at Capernaum also had an "epileptic" seizure. He was a member of the congregation listening to Jesus teaching in the synagogue.

> Now there was a man in the synagogue possessed by an unclean spirit. He shrieked, "What do you want with us, Jesus of Nazareth? Have you come to destroy us? I know who you are—the Holy One of God!" Jesus rebuked him: "Be silent," he said, "and come out of him." And the unclean spirit threw the man into convulsions and with a loud cry left him. (The

---

*Biblical translation requires emphasis on accuracy and readability. Therefore, words vary with emphasis as well as with manuscripts used in translation.

congregation were dumbfounded and noted that) "when he gives orders even the unclean spirits submit" (Mark 1:23–28).

Again, the parallel version adds a fragment. We learn that the devil after throwing the man down in front of the people left him without doing him any harm. This no doubt refers to the absence of injury to the tongue or bodily parts occasioned by the fall (Luke 4:33–36).

Some remarked that the illness of Apostle Paul cannot be diagnosed with certainty as epilepsy. Paul complained of a thorn in his flesh: "I was given a sharp pain in my body which came as Satan's messenger to bruise me; this was to save me from being unduly elated" (II Corinthians 12:7). He was glad that the Galatians did not spit before him to express their contempt as was done toward epileptics: "And you resisted any temptation to show scorn or disgust at the state of my poor body" (Galatians 4:14). On the road to Damascus a light flashed from the sky around him and he fell to the ground and heard a voice speak. He also replied to the voice. When he got up and opened his eyes he could not see; he was blind for 3 days and took no food or drink. Ananias later placed his hands on Paul and spoke to him. Consequently he regained his sight, was baptized, and took food (Acts 9:3–19). Some of the essential features of a seizure, such as involuntary movements, are missing. Some authors have interpreted this event in terms of conversion (Kaufman, 1964), probably more likely than an epileptic seizure, given the duration of the blindness, and prompt recovery after comforting.

Shakespeare

Epilepsy not only had been called "the sacred disease" by the ancients but also has become more commonly referred to as "the falling sickness" (Friedlander, 1963). The affection of the Roman Emperor Caesar is so described by Shakespeare:

> Casca: He *fell* down in the market-place, and *foamed at the mouth*, and was *speechless*.
> Brutus: 'Tis very like—he has the falling-sickness.
> Cassius: No, Caesar hath it not; but you, and I, and honest Casca, we have the falling-sickness.
> Casca: I know not what you mean by that; but, I am sure, Caesar fell down.
> Brutus: What said he when he came unto himself?
> Casca: When he came to himself again, he said, if he had done or said anything amiss, he desired their worships to think it was his *infirmity*.

(Julius Caesar, Act 1)

Shakespeare often referred to epilepsy and its manifestations:

> Iago: My lord is fallen into an epilepsy; this is his second fit—he had one yesterday.
>
> Cassio: Rub him about the temples.
>
> Iago: No, forbear: The lethargy must have his quiet course; if not he foams at mouth, and by and by breaks out to savage madness; Look! he stirs .... Do you withdraw yourself a little while, he will recover straight.

(Othello, Act IV)

Sherlock Holmes

Seizures and hysteria or malingering are mentioned on several occasions in the Sherlock Holmes series written by the physician, Arthur Conan Doyle. By far the most interesting of seizures concerns Sherlock Holmes in *The Reigate Squires*. We have Watson's description:

> ... [his] face had suddenly assumed the most dreadful expression. His eyes rolled upwards, his features writhed in agony, and with a suppressed groan, he dropped on his face upon the ground. Horrified by the sudden and severity of the attack, we carried him into the kitchen where he laid back in a large chair and breathed heavily for several minutes.

In the story, Holmes' "seizure" had been a trick devised to avert attention from a suspected criminal and had successfully fooled even Dr. Watson,, who conceded, "... speaking professionally, it was admirably done."

In "The Resident Patient," Dr. Percy Trevelyan, the author of a monograph on obscure nervous lesions, described a patient who suffered recurrent spells described thus:

> He ceased to give any answer at all to my inquiries and on my turning towards him, I was shocked to see that he was sitting bolt upright in his chair staring at me with a perfectly bland and rigid face.

The doctor was able to tell this was not a true seizure because the patient's pulse, temperature, muscle tone and reflexes were unchanged. The patient, feigning illness to gain entrance to Dr. Trevelyan's house, simulated a complex partial seizure, rather than a generalized tonic-clonic seizure, a more common form of hysterical seizure in Victorian years.

References

Beeson. B.B. Jean Martin Charcot. *Ann. Med. Hist.* (Ser. 1) 10:126, 1928.
Brain, Sir R., and Harvey, W. Neurologist. *Br. Med. J.* 2:899, 1959.

Brazier, M.A.B. The EEG in epilepsy: An historical note. *Epilepsia* 1:328, 1950.

Brazier, M.A.B. Richard Caton: The discoverer of the electrical activity of the brain. *Spike Wave* 7:12, 1958.

Bright, R. Fatal epilepsy, from suppuration between the dura mater and arachnoid, in consequence of blood having been effused in that situation. *Guy Hosp. Rep.* 1:36, 1836.

Brim, C.J. Paralysis in the Old Testament: A treatise on some of the neurological observations recorded in the Bible by ancient Hebrew prophets. *J. Nerv. Ment. Dis.* 97:656, 1943.

Broadbent, W.H. Hughlings Jackson as pioneer in nervous physiology and pathology. *Brain* 26:305, 1903.

Brown-Séquard, C.E. Récherches expérimentales sur la production d'une affection convulsive épileptiforme, à la suite de lésions de la möelle épinière. *Arch. Gen. Med.* (Ser. 5) 7:142, 1856.

Brown-Séquard, C.E. *Course of Lectures on the Physiology and Pathology of the Central Nervous System.* Collins, Philadelphia, 1860.

Bucher, H. W. *Tissot und sein Traete des nerfs, ein Beitrag zur Medizengeschiehte der Schweizerischen Aufklärung.* Juris, Zurich, 1958.

Calmeil, L.F. De L'épilepsie, étudiée sous le rapport de son siège et de son influence sur la production de l'alienation mentale. These de Paris, 1824.

Cooke, J. *A Treatise on Nervous Disease.* Longman, London, 1820–1823.

Copeland, J. *Of the Causes, Nature and Treatment of the Forms, Seats Complications, and Morbid Relations of Paralytic and Apoplectic Diseases.* Lea and Blanchard, Philadelphia, 1850.

Courvelle, C.B. Epilepsy in mythology, legend and folk tale. *Bull. Los Angeles Neurol. Soc.* 16:213, 1951.

Critchley, M. Hughlings Jackson: The man and the early days of the National Hospital. *Proc. R. Soc. Med.* 53:613, 1960.

Delasiauve, L.J.R. *Traite de l'Epilepsie: Histoire, Traitement, Médecine, Légale.* Masson, Paris, 1854.

Drabkin, I. E. Caelius Aurelianus: On Acute Diseases and on Chronic Disease. University of Chicago, Chicago, 1950.

Esquirol, J.E.D. *Des Maladies Mentalis.* Paris, J.B., Baillière, 1838.

Flourens MJP. *Recherches sur les Propriétés et les Fonctions du Système Nerveux, dans les Animaux Vertébrés.* Crevot, Paris, 1824.

Freud, S. Charcot. In *Collected Works of Sigmund Freud,* edited by Jones, E. Books, Inc., New York, 1959.

Friedlander, W.J. Shakespeare on epilepsy. *Boston Med. Q.* 14:113, 1963.

Fulton, J.F. *Neurophysiological Backgrounds of Modern Clinical Neurology* (with addition from J. Mt. Sinai Hosp., vol. 22, 1956) C.P. Rollins, New Haven, 1956.

Fulton, J.F. History of focal epilepsy. *Int. J. Neurol.* 1:21, 1959.

Fulton, J.F., and Cushing, H. A bibliographical study of the Galvani and the Aldini writing on animal electricity. *Ann. Sci.* 1:237, 1936.

Galen, C. De tremore, palpitatione, convulsione et rigore. Edited and translated from the Greek, by Kühn, G.G. Opera, 7:584 Lipsiae 1824.

Galen, C. Advice for an epileptic boy. (Translated from the Greek by Owsei Temkin). *Bull. Hist. Med.* 2:129, 1934.

Galvani, A.L. De viribus electricitatis in motu musculari commentarius cum Joannis Aldini dessertatione et notis: Accesserunt epistolae ad animals electricitatis theoriam pertinentes. Mutine, apud Societatem typographicam, 1792.

Garrison, F.H. Charcot: For his centenary (November 25, 1925). *Int. Clin.* (ser. 35) 4:244, 1925.

Garrison, F.H. *An Introduction to the History of Medicine,* ed. 4. Saunders, Philadelphia, 1929.

Ginzberg, R. Three years with Hans Berger (1873–1942): A contribution to his biography. *J. Hist. Med.* 4:361, 1949.

Gowers, W.R. *Epilepsy and Other Chronic Convulsive Diseases.* J & A Churchill, London, 1881.

Greenblatt, S. The major influences on the early life and work of John Hughlings Jackson. *Bull. Hist. Med. 39*:346, 1965.

Hall, M. *Synopsis of Cerebral and Spinal Seizures of Inorganic Origin and of Paroxysmal Form as a Class, and of Their Pathology as Involved in the Structures and Actions of the Neck.* J. Mallett, London, 1851.

Hall, M. *Synopsis of Apoplexy and Epilepsy: With Observations on the Trachelismus, Larynigismus and Tracheotomy, and the Proposal for a Hospital for Epileptics.* J. Mallett, London, 1852.

Havens, L.L. Charcot and hysteria. *J. Nerv. Ment. Dis. 141*:505–516, 1966.

Haymaker, W.E. *The Founders in Neurology: One Hundred and Thirty-Three Biographical Sketches.* Thomas, Springfield, IL, 1953.

Heberden, W. Epilepsy, head-ache, palsy and apoplexy, and St. Vitus dance. In *Commentaries on the History and Cure of Diseases.* T. Payne, London, 1802.

Hunter, R., and MacAlpine, I. William Harvey: His neurological and psychiatric observations. *J. Hist. Med. 12*:126, 1957.

Huxley, A. *The Devils of London.* Harper & Row, New York, 1957.

Ilberg, G. Das neurologisch-psyshistrische Wissen und Können des Aretäus von Kappadokien. *Z. Gesamte Neurol. 86*: 227, 1923.

Jefferson, G. The prodromes to cortical localization. *J. Neurol. Neurosurg. Psychiatry 16*: 59, 1953.

Kaufmann, J.C.D. Neuropathology in the Bible. *S. Afr. Med. J. 38*:748, 788, 805, 1964.

Lennox, W.G. John of Gaddesden on epilepsy. *Ann. Med. Hist.* (ser 3) *1*:283, 1939.

Lennox, W.G. Bernard of Gordon on epilepsy. *Ann. Med. Hist.* (ser 3) *3*:372, 1941.

Lennox, W.G. The centenary of bromides. *N. Engl. J. Med. 256*:887, 1957.

McHenry, L.C. *Garrison's History of Neurology.* Charles C Thomas, Springfield, IL, 1969.

McIntyre, N. Robert Bentley Todd. *Kings Coll. Hosp. Gaz. 35*:79, 184, 1956.

Maisonneuve, J.G.F. *Recherches et Observations sur l'Épilepsie.* Présentées à l'école de Médecine de Paris. Paris, 1804.

Major, R.H. Hippocrate et la neurologie. *World Neurol. 2*:654, 1961.

Moreau, J.J. *De l'Étiologie de l'Épilepsie et des Indications que l'Étude des Causes peut Fournir.* Baillière, Paris, 1854.

Penfield, W.G. Hippocratic preamble: The brain and intelligence. In *The History and Philosphy of Knowledge of the Brain and Its Functions,* edited by Poynter, F.N.L. Blackwell, Oxford, 1958.

Portal, A. *Observations sur la Nature et le Traitement de l'Épilepsie.* J. B. Baillière, Paris, 1827.

Prichard, J.C. *A Treatise on Disease of the Nervous System.* Underwood, London, 1822.

Prince, M. American neurology of the past: Neurology of the future. *N. Nerv. Ment. Dis. 42*:445, 1915.

Reynolds, J.R. *Epilepsy: Its Symptoms, Treatment and Relation to Other Chronic Convulsive Diseases.* John Churchill, London, 1861.

Rhomberg, M.H. *A Manual of the Nervous Diseases of Man,* edited and translated by Sieveking H. Syndenham Society, London, 1853.

Richer: *Etudes Cliniques sur la Grande Hystérie.* Delahaye et Zeerosnier, Paris, 1885.

Riese, W. The sources of Jacksonian neurology. *J. Nerv. Ment. Dis. 124*:125, 1956.

Schroeder van der Kolk, J.L.C. *Bau und Functionen der Medulla spinalis und oblongata, und nächste Ursache und rationelle Behandlung der Epilepsie.* F. Vieweg und Sohn, Braunschweig, 1859.

Sieveking, Sir E.H. *On Epilepsy and Epileptiform Seizures: Their Causes, Pathology and Treatment.* John Churchill, London, 1858.

Storch, E.P., and Storch, T.J.C. Arnold of Villanova on epilepsy. *Ann. Med. Hist. 10*:251, 1938.

Temkin, O. The doctrine of epilepsy in the Hippocratic writings. *Bull. Hist. Med. 1*:277, 1933.

Temkin, O. Views on epilepsy in the Hippocratic period. *Bull. Hist. Med. 1*:41, 1933.

Temkin, O. Epilepsy in an anonymous Greek work on acute and chronic diseases. *Bull. Hist. Med. 4*:137, 1936.

Temkin, O. The Falling-Sickness: A History of Epilepsy from the Greeks to the Beginnings of Modern Neurology. Baltimore, Johns Hopkins, 1945.

Temkin, O. Research on epilepsy before Hughlings Jackson. In *Epilepsy*. Publication of the Association for Research of Nervous and Mental Diseases, vol. 26. Williams & Wilkins, Baltimore, 1947.

Throckmorten, T.B. Frances X. Dercum: Physician, teacher and philosopher. *J. Nerv. Ment. Dis.* 96:529, 1942.

Tissot, S.A.A.D. *Traité des Nerfs et de Leurs Maladies.* Didot, Paris, 1770–1780.

Todd, R.B. *Clinical Lectures on Paralysis, Certain Diseases of the Brain, and Other Affections of the Nervous System.* Lindsay & Blakiston, Philadelphia, 1855.

Walshe, Sir F. Contributions of John Hughlings Jackson to neurology: A brief introduction to his teachings. *Arch. Neurol.* 5:119, 1961.

SECTION 1 # MEDICAL AND NEUROLOGICAL ASPECTS

Chapter 2 Recognition and Diagnostic Aspects of Nonepileptic Seizures

DONALD F. SCOTT, F.R.C.P., D.P.M.

The distinction between genuine epileptic seizures and pseudoseizures often is made without difficulty. This is particularly the case when the pseudoseizure mimics a true convulsive attack, whose pattern is usually unequivocal. In contrast the distinction can be difficult when the episode approximates a partial complex seizure (Remick and Wada, 1979), a temporal lobe attack for which there is a wide differential diagnosis (Scott, 1978 a). There are problems in the diagnosis of "true" epilepsy itself when a faint leads to a definite seizure because of the resulting cerebral hypoxia. Such conditions will not be covered here and little attention will be paid to such phenomena as episodes of rage or hyperventilation attacks, described elsewhere in this volume.

The present chapter is largely based on personal observation and that of physician colleagues interested in the problems of pseudoseizures. An attempt is made to bring these observations together in the light of the literature, which although considerable is rather patchy. It is hoped that what follows will prove of value in a difficult diagnostic area, one encountered by every doctor dealing with patients who have an attack disorder but often causing puzzlement. The chapter is divided into the following sections: the occurrence of pseudoseizures, antecedent factors, observation of the attacks themselves, use of EEG in diagnosis, and the attitude and experience of physicians. Finally, there is a brief review of a series of London Hospital patients who developed pseudoseizures and who had previously been diagnosed as having true epilepsy.

OCCURRENCE

The recognition of pseudoseizures is of importance as they are not infrequent in neurological practice. Any absolute figures about occurrence in relation to genuine epilepsy are difficult to obtain. However, if a rather specific group is studied, namely those patients in whom there is no doubt about the original diagnosis of epilepsy and who then developed pseudoseizures, they are found in our experience to be a common cause of admission to the hospital for reassessment of an attack disorder. A tentative figure for the occurrence in relation to outpatient attendance of epileptic patients in general would be about 5%; however, because of the frequency of attacks in the individual patient and the difficulty in diagnosis and in management, the pseudoseizure represents a significant problem.

ANTECEDENT FACTORS

The previous medical history is often the first feature which leads the physician to consider epilepsy as the cause of the patient's episodic disorder. Evidence strongly indicative of brain damage at birth and subsequent head injuries are two such factors, while a history suggestive of encephalitis or other neurological disorders in which subsequent epilepsy is known as a sequela may be similarly interpreted. Of interest is the comment of Standage (1975) who noted an excess of organic pathology in pseudoseizure patients, and Whitlock (1967) has reported this for hysteria patients in general.

Particular significance is often attached to the patient's account of his/her epilepsy, which may initially sway the physician into believing that this is the only diagnosis in spite of the fact that it is well-known that pseudoseizures may occur in patients with a definite history of a seizure disorder. Such a combination has been appreciated at least since the latter half of the 19th century (see Gowers, 1885, for example). More recently Standage (1975) has drawn attention to this problem, and Roy (1977) has given detailed pointers for help in the establishment of the true diagnosis.

It is important in management to establish what other physicians have previously thought. Their case notes should be obtained and carefully reviewed where possible. Reliance should not be placed entirely on the account of the patient or indeed of the relatives. In all instances in which pseudoseizures are suspected, consideration of psychiatric factors is of great importance (Roy, 1977; Guberman, 1980/81). Some of these may have emerged from the earlier case papers; although, as with many other features, they do not provide an absolute distinction between true seizures and pseudoseizures, they usually provide strong evidence for one or the other of these diagnoses. Evidence of depressive illness and suicidal attempts, marital disharmony and difficulty in managing children, misuse of drugs and alcohol all tend to point in the direction of pseudoseizures. On the other hand, depressive illness has been shown by Betts and colleagues (1976) to be one of the most common causes of psychiatric referral in those who have genuine epilepsy.

Personality factors must be assessed. The hysterical or the inadequate personality may suggest that pseudoseizures are likely, and stigmata of minor suicidal attempts, for example, numerous small scars on the front of the wrists, may give a clue. Marital and employment history are important factors to weigh but may be difficult to obtain initially. Exposure of the patient to seizures at home or at work is a valuable piece of evidence. Also pseudoseizures are not by any means the prerogative of the uneducated and unsophisticated (Liske and Forster, 1964), as any physician will be able to recount in long experience of difficult attack disorders; indeed, nurses and paramedical personnel are often overrepresented in this group. One problem frequently encountered is the drowsy and drugged patient on initial referral. This may have resulted from either illicit drug taking or ingestion of alcohol, but often it is because the diagnosis of a true seizure disorder has been made, by others, and sedative anticonvulsant medication has been given. In such a state, diagnosis may be difficult.

OBSERVATION OF THE ATTACKS

The differences between hysterical attacks and true seizures have been reviewed by Scott (1978 b) and by Roy in Chapter 8 of this book. What follows highlights the main difficulties. The state of the patient when first seen may be perplexing not only because of a possible postictal condition. The patient may have his or her face turned away from the light and display little coherent response. This type of picture may be seen after either definite seizures or pseudoseizures. One of the problems is the interpretation of noises emitted by the patient prior to or during the attack, whether heard by the physician or reported by observers. Such sounds may be a form of ictal iteration as noted in some forms of partial complex seizures or the involuntary accompaniment at the start of a convulsion. In neither case is there any sustained organized speech.

The motor movements affecting all four limbs may appear, likewise, as the clonic phase of a true seizure. However, preceding tonic manifestations are in our experience uncommon in pseudoseizures. In these cases, detailed examination of the apparent clonic jerks indicates their random pseudopurposive nature; for example, they may occur initially in one arm and follow in the opposite leg—difficult to explain on a neurophysiological basis. The semipurposive nature of the motor phenomena, such as kicking, pushing and slapping rather than mere jerking with changing rhythmicity, usually lead the physician to believe that he is dealing with a pseudoseizure. However, partial complex seizures are remarkably variable in their manifestations; a variety of different automatisms occur which may render the physician in a quandary as to the nature of the underlying disorder, even if he is fortunate to examine one or even many such attacks firsthand. There may be, in the partial seizure, a marked difference between the motor phenomena on one side compared with those on the other side, e.g., rubbing of the leg or patting of the hair with the right hand while the left hand is still. In these instances, interpretation of which hemisphere is "firing" can be problematical, but usually adversive components are helpful in that the head and eyes turn away from the hemisphere showing the epileptic discharge.

Traditional methods of determining whether a seizure is genuine or not, such as studying the eyes or eliciting the plantar responses, may not be entirely conclusive. The pseudoseizure patient is usually said to screw up his or her eyes and turn away when examination is attempted, but resistance to this maneuver may also be found in the true postictal confusional state. Usually the plantar responses are regarded as diagnostic, but Hammond (1948) has noted an extensor plantar response in a patient who was almost certainly having a pseudoseizure. Opisthotonic posture occurs in both true seizures and pseudoseizures, and salivation likewise occurs in both. All these features may trap even the wary doctor.

There are three other phenomena which are generally regarded as making a clear distinction between the true seizure and the pseudoseizure: tongue biting, incontinence and injury. It is generally taught and accepted that these *never* occur in patients with pseudoseizures. This is a gross oversimplification and may lead to an incorrect diagnosis. In our recent experience, incontinence (Jasper, 1963; Toone and Roberts, 1979) has been a common manifestation and bruising, injury and tongue biting have also been observed, although less frequently.

Two personal examples, both young women, may be cited here. One patient who had personally been confidently diagnosed as having status epilepticus showed a large calcified hematoma on the forehead as a result of falls. After a long and stormy course of inpatient care during which anticonvulsants were completely withdrawn (Niedermeyer et al., 1970), under the cover of placebo, it became clear that all the attacks at that stage were without doubt pseudoseizures.

The second, likewise a complicated case, came into the doctor's office as another patient was being interviewed. When asked to wait outside, she simply keeled over backwards, hitting her head on a metal radiator and sustaining concussion and severe occipital laceration. The latter incident raises the matter of the distinction between malingering (Naish, 1979) and the hysterical pseudoseizure, a complex gray area but one that must be borne in mind by the physician presented with patients who display attack disorders.

The duration of the attack is a matter which requires careful consideration. Genuine seizures usually have a fairly discrete and stereotyped form lasting at most a few minutes, although a series may occur occasionally. These may prove difficult to distinguish from the pseudoseizure in which apparent disturbance of consciousness with motor concomitants may persist for half an hour to several hours. Then the patient may be labelled as having status epilepticus and treated as such. The frequency of the attacks is also important. The fact that many are observed during a 24-hour period is obviously worrying to the physician and will sway him, even in the absence of full diagnosis, toward vigorous drug treatment. However, when the attacks occur in the home situation, in the presence of relatives or dramatically during the hospital visiting hour, the doctor must think again.

Genuine seizures may recur very frequently, and then are usually associated with a degree of obtundation; rarely can such a patient carry on a detailed and coherent conversation, in contrast to the pseudoseizure patient to whom large doses of medication have not been given. Consideration should also be given to attacks in bed, in the street, or when the patient is on his own. All of these tend to suggest a genuine epileptic disorder, although exceptions may be encountered; a recent personal case almost certainly had pseudoseizures in bed at night. Of course, the "experienced" patient may know that the physician considers an audience to be important in establishing the diagnosis of pseudoseizures and may simply lie in relation to whether or not attacks occur when she is alone.

Toone and Roberts (1979) drew attention to the fact that pseudoseizure patients may have serial attacks or what amounts to status epilepticus. In a group from the London Hospital (more details later), 2 or possibly 3 of 32 patients had such frequent attacks that they were treated as though they had status. This was quite definite in 2 because the documentation was complete, but in the other patient status epilepticus had not been documented, a feature that often presents difficulties in assessing pseudoseizure patients in other respects. The two patients both developed the condition when under the care of other doctors, i.e., not their regular physicians, who were not aware of the complex nature of the disorder presented. One patient when on holiday abroad was admitted to an intensive therapy unit and had a tracheostomy. The problem of management here, as in other cases, was compounded by the fact that anticonvulsant drugs had been given in large doses, leading, firstly, to problems in establishing the diagnosis and, secondarily, to respiratory difficulties. Hence, the diagnosis of status was made and apparently appropriate treatment was instituted with intravenous medication. The other patient absconded from the care of her usual physician and subsequently was admitted in apparent status to a hospital some distance away. In this instance, a telephone conversation put the attending doctor's mind at rest and the proposed continuation of a heavy program of intravenous drugs was stopped and recovery ensued. This was hastened by confronting the apparently unconscious patient with the information about her past history received in the telephone call.

ACTIONS OF THE OBSERVER

What should the observer do if confronted with a patient having an attack which could be a pseudoseizure? Traditionally, a slap on the face, making a loud noise and dousing with cold water have all been tried, but does the response to these "treatments" indicate the nature of the attack? If the maneuvers are effective and abort the attack, what does it indicate? Again the usual view would be that the attack was not a genuine seizure. Such a conclusion is erroneous; for example, sensory stimuli of the type mentioned above will stop a petit mal attack and block the concomitant 3 cycle per second generalized spike and wave discharge in the EEG. Once again, we find that the observation of one particular feature or phenomenon is not completely diagnostic.

Another question concerns the induction of seizures. A considerable proportion of patients with epilepsy say that they have the ability, for example, by thinking of a particular idea or by placing a limb in a certain posture, to elicit (or indeed stop) development of a fit. Hence, confronted with this history from a patient, the physician may feel that the seizure is in fact of genuine type. This is in our experience not always the case and, as Liske and Forster (1964) pointed out, it is unwise to make a diagnosis of a true seizure disorder in a patient who has an *unusual* attack triggered by an *unusual* stimulus. They quote as an example "eating a piece of cheese." To be certain that the attack is a genuine form of reflex epilepsy, EEG monitoring is necessary. Even this is not straightforward because patients with a genuine reflex seizure problem may, in the laboratory situation, be unable to precipitate an attack even though appropriate stimuli ("internal," of the sort mentioned above, or "external" as in the case of reading or musicogenic epilepsy) are presented.

In summary, do not be overimpressed by traditional teaching about individual phenomena, such as incontinence, as indicating clearly that the episodic disorder is definitely epilepsy. Interpretation of observations made in these patients, like the history, may need to be assessed with extreme care.

THE USE OF EEG IN DIAGNOSIS

The use of EEG in monitoring patients during triggering procedures forms a small part of the value of the technique, the main aspects of which have been briefly reported by Moffett and Scott (1981), in particular the interseizure record may be confusing to the referring physician if neither he nor the encephalographer is clear about the facts of the case. A considerable proportion of patients who have pseudoseizures may have had epilepsy in the past and their tracings then frequently show clear-cut abnormalities in terms of spikes, sharp waves, localized or generalized complexes or all these forms of epileptiform discharge in combination. When the features are localized there is usually a preponderance of abnormality in the temporal areas, and there may be a side difference which does not always correspond to the generality of partial complex seizure patients, in whom left hemisphere abnormalities are most frequent (Currie et al., 1971). Bursts of spike and wave which may be almost typical in type are very infrequent.

Taking these interseizure encephalographic features at their face value, a referring physician would almost certainly conclude, and wrongly so, that he is dealing with genuine epilepsy. The important point here is to consider the amount of EEG abnormality in relation to the reported seizure frequency. Generally with the pseudoseizure case there are only occasional discharges (Niedermeyer et al, 1970) in the presence of very frequent attacks. In such instances, particular emphasis should be given to the background activity. The whole tracing may have a well-organized appearance, and the frequency of the alpha elements may be within the normal range. Only small amounts of slow activity will be present, such elements being seen in brief episodes particularly over the temporal regions.

The EEG picture here may have been altered by the administration of drugs (Toone and Roberts, 1979), excessive fast components when benzodiazepines have been given, or slowing of the tracing when large quantities of this or other anticonvulsant medication have been administered. This latter is a confusing factor but, in general, with frequent genuine seizures the alpha rhythm is usually at the low end of the normal range or in the upper theta band, being disorganized and interspersed with large quantities of slow activity.

Sometimes the EEG may be recorded during an actual attack. If this is the case, then positive evidence that this was a true seizure or a pseudoseizure can usually be determined with certainty (Aird, 1956; Liske and Forster, 1964). In the former, spiking or other discharges may be seen to commence locally and spread widely. Attenuation of the alpha rhythm may have preceded this, as an aura develops. Following the attack, flattening of background elements will be seen. Then, almost invariably, slow activity appears and persists for many minutes and often hours afterward. The pseudoseizure pattern is generally different, although the alpha activity may be blocked during the attack itself; preceding it and within moments of cessation a well-organized alpha rhythm may appear. Muscle components can be confusing since they may be taken to be spikes of cerebral origin. The main point of distinction lies in careful examination of the seizure discharge: the spikes which form it tend to have a rhythmical nature rather than occurring in discrete bursts as is characteristic of muscle activity. This may appear first in bursts on one side of the head and then on the other or in a rather random fashion, quite uncharacteristic of the origin and spread of discharge if of the focal type or of the generalized seizure pattern starting suddenly.

It is important in these patients to review all the EEGs that can be obtained. Previous tracings may reveal pseudoseizures or true seizures that had been wrongly interpreted. Sleep records or tracings with additional leads such as sphenoidals (Remick and Wada, 1979) may be helpful, as may obtaining an EEG as soon after an attack as possible. When these methods fail to give the diagnosis, there are other more complex procedures available. The use of combined EEG monitoring and closed circuit television is one such and telemetry another. Ambulant monitoring with the subsequent examination of the taped EEG may also be helpful.

Recently, it has been suggested that biochemical tests may be helpful. For example, prolactin levels rise significantly after epileptic convulsions but not after hysterical ones (Trimble, 1978).

We have employed a simple EEG technique using the Cerebral Function Monitor (Prior et al., 1971). A single channel compressed EEG record is produced. The electrodes are applied to the scalp in the usual way and the leads connected to the apparatus on a trolley by the patient, who may either sit or lie throughout the monitoring procedure for hours or days. Discharges can be seen on the tracing when due to seizures (Prior, 1979). At other times, when the patient complains of an attack or when one is witnessed, the absence of electrical changes in the tracing can also be noted. The muscle activity appears in an additional channel, aiding diagnosis. These tracings can be most helpful in distinguishing between epileptic and nonepileptic seizures (Moffett and Scott, 1981).

Although the EEG revolutionized modern understanding of epilepsy and cerebral function, failure to recognize some of the normal variant patterns has led to a diagnosis of epilepsy in persons who by clinical criteria would not be considered to have epileptic disorders. As Maulsby (1979) indicated, the early years of the subject were largely spent in identifying sharp pointed waves in tracings, associating those with the subject's complaints, and concluding that the symptoms and EEG patterns were causally related. The obvious drawback in such an approach was the omission of control subjects who might have the same EEG pattern but lacked the same complaints. However, definite changes like spikes, sharp waves and spike and wave are very rare even in neurological patients in the absence of clinical epilepsy, of the order of 2% (Zivin and Marsan, 1968). Even if these findings are seen, a seizure disorder might correctly be expected to occur subsequently.

Several EEG features have been described which are quite distinctive in terms of voltage, their sudden manner of arising from the background activity, rhythmical qualities or sharp and pointed features, that is using the international definitions of paroxysmal (Chatrian et al., 1974). Some are of current interest, 6 per second spike and wave discharges (phantom spike and wave), 14 and 6 positive spikes (ctenoids or 14 and 6), the "psychomotor variant" pattern and small sharp spikes (SSS, benign epileptiform transients of sleep—BETS). These patterns which occur fairly frequently among normals are seen in patients with epilepsy (Maulsby, 1979; Reiher and Klass, 1968; Tharp, 1966). Some of these are sufficiently prominent in the EEG of patients who have fleeting or recurrent disorders of behavior or consciousness to present a problem of interpretation; this indicates that, as with other fields of medicine, rigid criteria should be abandoned. It is, nevertheless, a not infrequent experience in epilepsy clinics that an individual who has episodes which are truly syncopal attacks or who has hysterical attacks may have been erroneously diagnosed as epileptic in the past on the basis of an EEG recording which contained, for example, 14 and 6 per second positive spikes or 6 Hz spike wave patterns or other types of unusual disturbance.

In summary, for the difficult case it is worth pursuing electroencephalographic procedures well beyond the performance of repeated routine recordings, and it is also important to be aware of truly normal patterns which have wave forms or voltages which might mimic those characteristic of epileptic seizures.

THE ATTITUDE OF THE PHYSICIAN

When considering a pseudoseizure, the physician must approach the problem without undue bias, a point made by Lennox and Lennox (1960). Obviously, experience and observation of many such patients are of great benefit, but sometimes the notes of the naive may yield a clue to the true diagnosis because they are not clouded by expectations of what should or should not be seen. It is quite true that the bizarre theatrical performance of some patients is there for all to see, as is the stereotyped pattern of the convulsion. However, complex partial seizures can be difficult to distinguish from pseudoseizures (Johnson and Lewis, 1976), and all one's faculties are required to make the correct diagnosis. Two further points: Even the highly experienced and trained observer may not be able to make the diagnosis (Toone and Roberts, 1979), although usually it becomes clear with the passage of time and repeated observation and reports of relatives and others. Nevertheless, most physicians will have to admit that in a few patients seen over many years, there is still a lingering doubt as to the true nature of their attack disorder.

One of the difficulties concerns the literature. It is sparse and patchy, partly because there is lack of any absolute criteria as to whether the disorder seen is a true seizure or a pseudoseizure condition. Physicians are apparently loath to talk about this matter at meetings or to write articles. The reason is self-evident, the hearer or the reader can simply dismiss the evidence saying he believes the other diagnosis is the correct one. So far the term "hysterical" has largely been avoided but there is, of course, no doubt that this is the rubric under which many pseudoseizures have to be classified, and certainly "hysterical" is a term associated with a considerable emotional overlay for patient and physician alike. It is a complex subject and its psychopathological aspects and conceptualizations have recently been usefully reviewed by Merskey (1979). Although hysterical manifestations were more common in the western countries in an earlier century, they still occur and this label is perhaps underused partly because of the observations of Slater (1965) in his classical paper indicating that patients who had been confidently diagnosed as having an hysterical disorder subsequently revealed organic disease.

From a diagnostic point of view, malingering (Naish, 1979) and simulated seizures must not be excluded from consideration. One example must suffice, the patient in her mid twenties was a nurse. She was admitted because of attacks which had been confidently passed as genuine. They occurred in a series almost amounting to status and the temperature was then noted to be elevated. She had scars of previous injuries, but there was little in her own or the family background which aided diagnosis. It was an astute ward sister's observation which unravelled the problem. The saliva in the corners of the mouth after a series of fits she noted was somewhat suspicious in color and when tested for blood was found to be negative. It subsequently transpired that the patient had filled her mouth with black-current syrup prior to the attack, a drink favored by many hospital patients. This was the first clue and then a search of personal possessions revealed a series of thermometers which could be adjusted appropriately. Patients with this type of disorder tend to be paraparetic and some could be placed in the category of the Munchausen syndrome. They are, fortunately, rare but most physicians will encounter at least one in their lifetime of practice.

THE LONDON HOSPITAL SERIES

This chapter has been largely and of necessity anecdotal since statistical information is not readily available in such cases. However, we have a series of 32 patients who without doubt had been diagnosed as having a true seizure disorder in the past and then attended with pseudoseizures. They show the general characteristics of other series. There were 30 women and only 2 men; their average age was 35 years, with a range from 16 to 55 years. The upper end should be noted as Ferriss (1959) has reported that pseudoseizure disorders may commence in the 50s. The duration of epilepsy was on average 9.5 years. The most characteristic pattern was a relapsing and remitting course. The prognosis for the individual admissions or attendance when seizures had rapidly accelerated in frequency was good: they would subside spontaneously with general supportive care and attention to any stressful factors in the environment. A few patients ran a more malignant course and required institutional care. All had bulky case notes and a long series of EEGs. These showed abnormality in virtually all instances but with a markedly fluctuating pattern, related partly to the incidence of genuine seizures and to drug treatment. Management in a few of the patients was very difficult but became somewhat easier when a confident diagnosis of pseudoseizures had been made. Unfortunately even when it was clear that the basic diagnosis in these patients was psychiatric, formal help by the psychiatrist was often refused.

CONCLUSION

The diagnosis of pseudoseizure disorder requires all the skill of the physician. He must carefully evaluate the history obtained by himself and his staff as well as assess the case records gleaned from other hospitals. It is when the patient is first seen without benefit of previous information that greatest difficulty is encountered. Awareness of the various forms of the pseudoseizure that are taken is essential, bearing in mind that the categorical statements such as "incontinence never occurs" should be disregarded. In the long run, detailed observation is the most helpful means of clinching the diagnosis although intensive EEG investigations can prove valuable. If a confident diagnosis of a pseudoseizure is made, then anticonvulsants should be greatly reduced or totally withdrawn. The physician should not be overconfident in his initial assessment, bearing in mind that many expert observers have been misled and that it may only be in the course of prolonged surveillance that the true diagnosis is finally established.

ACKNOWLEDGMENTS

The author is grateful to Dr. R. A. Henson, Dr. A. Ridley, and Dr. M. Swash, neurologists at the London Hospital, for rekindling an interest in this difficult subject and for permission to report briefly findings which will be published in detail elsewhere.

References

Aird, R.B. *Epileptic Seizures*, edited by Green, J.R., and Steelman, H.F. Williams & Wilkins, Baltimore, 1956.

Betts, T.A., Merskey, H., and Pond, D.A. Psychiatry. In *A Textbook of Epilepsy*, edited by Laidlaw, T., and Richens, A. Churchill, Livingstone, London, 1976.

Currie, S., Heathfield, K.W.G., Henson, R.A., and Scott, D.F. Clinical course and progress of temporal lobe epilepsy. *Brain* 94:173–190, 1971.

Ferriss, G.S. The recognition of nonepileptic seizures. *South. Med. J.* 52:1557–1567, 1959.

Gowers, W.R. *Epilepsy*. 1885, reprinted by Dover Press, New York, 1969.

Guberman, A. Hysterical pseudoseizures: Differential diagnosis from epilepsy. In *Perspectives in Epilepsy*. British Epilepsy Association, Crowthorne, Berks, England, 1980/81.

Hammond, R.D. Simulated epilepsy: Report of a case. *Arch. Neurol. Psychiatry* 60:327–328, 1948.

Jaspers, K. *General Psychopathology*, translated by Hoenig, J., and Hamilton, M.W. Manchester University Press, Manchester, 1963.

Johnson, S.M., and Lewis, J.A. The hysterical seizure. *Am. J. EEG Technol.* 16:23–29, 1976.

Lennox, W.G., and Lennox, M.A. *Epilepsy and Related Disorders*. Little, Brown, Boston, 1960.

Liske, E., and Forster, F.M., Pseudoseizures: A problem in diagnosis and management of epileptic patients. *Neurology* 41:41–49, 1964.

Maulsby, R.L. EEG patterns of uncertain diagnostic significance. In *Current Practice of Clinical Electroencephalography*, edited by Klass, D.W., and Daly, D.D. Raven Press, New York, 1979, pages 411–420.

Merskey, H. *The Analysis of Hysteria*. Bailliere Tindall, London, 1979.

Moffett, A., and Scott, D.F. The EEG in the diagnosis of hysterical attacks in patients with epilepsy. *Electroencephalogr. Clin. Neurophysiol.* 1981, in press.

Naish, J.M. Problems of deception in medical practice. *Lancet* 2:139–142, 1979.

Niedermeyer, E., Blumer, D., Holscher, E., and Walker, B.A. Classical hysterical seizures facilitated by anticonvulsant toxicity. *Psychiatr. Clin.* 3:71–84, 1970.

Prior, P.F. *Monitoring Cerebral Function.* Elsevier North Holland, Amsterdam, 1979.

Prior, P.F., Maynard, D.E., Sheaff, P.C., Simpson, B.R., Strunin, L., Weaver, E.J.M., and Scott, D.F. Monitoring cerebral function: Clinical experience with a new device for continuous recording of activity of the brain. *Br. Med. J.* 2:2051–2054, 1971.

Reiher, J., and Klass, D.W. Two common EEG patterns of doubtful clinical significance. *Med. Clin. North Am.* 52:933–940, 1968.

Remick, R. A., and Wada, J.A. Complex partial and pseudo-seizure disorders. *Am. J. Psychiatry* 136:320–323, 1979.

Roy, A. Hysterical fits, previously diagnosed as epilepsy. *Psychol. Med.* 7:271–273, 1977.

Scott, D.F. a. Temporal lobe epilepsy. *Br. J. Hosp. Med.* 22:178–187, 1978.

Scott, D.F. b. Psychiatric aspects of epilepsy. *Br. J. Psychiatry* 132:417–430, 1978.

Standage, K.F. The aetiology of hysterical seizures. *Can. Psychiatr. Assoc. J.* 20:67–73, 1975.

Tharp, B.R. The 6-per-second spike and wave complex. *Arch. Neurol.* 15:533–537, 1966.

Toone, B.K., and Roberts, J. Status epilepticus: An uncommon hysterical conversion syndrome. *J. Nerv. Ment. Dis.* 167:548–552, 1979.

Trimble, M.A. Serum prolactic in epilepsy and hysteria. *Br. Med. J.* 4:1682, 1978.

Whitlock, F.A. The aetiology of hysteria. *Acta Psychiatr. Scand.* 43:144–162, 1967.

Zivin, L., Ajmone-Marsan, C. Incidence and prognostic significance of epileptiform activity in the EEG in non-epileptic subjects. *Brain* 91:751–780, 1968.

Chapter 3 Syncope and Hyperventilation

TERRENCE L. RILEY, M.D.

Syncope and hyperventilation attacks are two causes of alterations of consciousness which are frequently mistaken for epilepsy. In their simplest, classic forms, both conditions should be easily distinguishable from seizures; however, both may cause a wide range of symptoms which may appear remarkably similar to seizures. Distinguishing between these events and epileptic seizures may be complicated by the fact that hyperventilation can actually precipitate seizures, and autonomic sequelae of seizures may, secondarily, lead to cardiac arrhythmias or syncope. The identification of both hyperventilation and syncope demands specific treatment; however, this identification does not exclude the possibility of coexistent epilepsy.

Syncope

Syncope, or fainting, is the abrupt loss of consciousness caused by brain hypoxia or hypoperfusion. The word "syncope" is derived from the Greek synkope or synkoptein, meaning to cut, chop, or break. Apparently the term followed an earlier view of "petite mort" or "small death" as a cause of sudden break of consciousness. Bichat (1805) introduced the fundamental concept that, "The primary seat of the ill in syncope is always the heart ... the brain that dies because it *fails to receive from the heart the fluid....*" Littre subsequently embellished this description to note that "momentary suspension or decrease in action of the heart," heart block or transient arrythmia, could result in syncope (in Gastaut, 1974). The epileptic seizure, an energy-consuming excessive neuronal discharge, is such a fundamentally different event that the two disturbances should be easily distinguished. The clinician's frequent grappling between "fit versus faint" attests to the frustrating difficulty of distinguishing the two types of spells. Gastaut (1974), while emphasizing crucial physiologic differences between faints and sei-

34

zures, confessed to the clinical similarities by referring to syncopal attacks as "generalized anoxic seizures." Gowers (1901) included syncope among the phenomena he called the "borderlands of epilepsy," believing there may be a common pathophysiology.

Although there are many different causes of syncope, few are completely isolated or momentary conditions. The predisposing factors persist long enough so that syncopal attacks tend to recur: either for years (as in micturition syncope) or at least during the duration of an underlying disease—for example, volume depletion. Stereotypy and recurrence are often suggestive of epilepsy. There are further similarities to epileptic seizures. Depending on the suddenness of onset, there may be a characteristic blurring or alteration of perception at the beginning of attacks, which may be interpreted as an "aura" or perceptual distortion in a complex partial seizure. If diminished perfusion during a syncopal attack lasts long enough to release cortical inhibition of brain stem postural and vestibular mechanisms, an apparent "convulsion" may result. For all these similarities, careful description or, preferably, direct observation is seldom possible and, since even the experienced observer may require physiologic information, detailed EKG and/or EEG monitoring are often necessary adjuncts.

The symptoms and sequence of syncopal attacks follow a rather stereotyped pattern, but the rapidity of the sequence may vary with the precipitant and the general vascular state of the individual and may be affected by an initial postural response.

PREMONITORY SYMPTOMS

If the precipitant leads only slowly to total loss of consciousness (for example, paroxysmal atrial tachycardia in a healthy adolescent), there may be sensations of general malaise, lightness, aeration, or levitation in the head—the stage Gastaut calls "lipothymia." During this phase, often called "presyncope" because of a common premonition of loss of consciousness, response times are sluggish, vision blurs, and there may be vestibular or acoustic symptoms such as vertigo, tinnitus, or sensation of echoes. The person may have a feeling of time suspension, euphoria, or even hallucinations. The vividness and complexity of the subjective experiences of lipothymia are dependent upon duration: slower onset allows for slower and more elaborate distortions of perception and consciousness. When the experiences are "dreamy," stereotyped or hallucinatory, they may particularly suggest "auras" or temporal lobe discharges of complex partial seizures. Concomitant peripheral manifestations of hyperventilation, if present, may embellish symptoms further and may mimic cortical recruitment phenomena of seizures. If pulse rate, cerebral perfusion pressure, and oxygen content are not improved within 3 seconds, complete loss of consciousness usually supervenes and the individual slowly slumps to the ground. This is an important distinguishing feature from generalized tonic-clonic convulsion which is more often accompanied by a dystonic contortion or a propulsive jerking to the floor. The slow, crumbling or slumping fall to the ground or furniture, which is probably the most important descriptive feature of syncopal attack, is the reason injury from the fall itself is uncommon with syncope. By contrast, facial or head injuries are common with propulsive or convulsive falls from seizures. When observed or sought in the history, the moment of the fall can usually distinguish "fit from faint." An exception is the "temporal lobe syncope," a slow syncope-like collapse caused by some temporal lobe seizures (Caffi, 1973). In syncopal spells the process is usually reversed within 10 seconds of falling to horizontal posture. Especially in vasodepressor states, improved cardiac filling leads to increased cardiac output, and cerebral perfusion is corrected within about 10 seconds; a few generalized clonic jerks may occur, followed by a tonic hyperextended posture. More commonly the tonic phase occurs first; during relaxation, there may be a few (rarely more than three or four in convulsive syncope) brief generalized clonic contractions.

Following a syncopal attack of 10 seconds or longer in duration, the person is often momentarily clouded but may feel weak or concerned about the episode for several minutes. Frequently there is a sensation of needing to void or defecate; nausea is particularly frequent. Momentarily increased secretion of antidiuretic hormone during the spell often causes oliguria for hours afterward. The severity of postsyncopal symptoms usually depends upon the duration of the loss of consciousness and is more pronounced after convulsive spells. A person may be so fatigued, uncomfortable, or confused that he or she prefers to sleep or rest for an hour or longer. The constellation of premonitory mental symptoms, loss of consciousness, clonic shaking of all extremities, and then a postictal sleepiness may all sound very much like a seizure.

CONVULSIVE SYNCOPE

In syncope, when the duration of cerebral hypoperfusion is extended, there may be actual convulsive stiffening or repetitive generalized shaking movements which are scarcely distinguishable from postures or clonic movements of seizures. This is a common phenomenon among military populations. When a soldier standing for a long time faints and his cohorts hold him erect to escape detection, the improved cardiac return from falling to a horizontal position is avoided. The result often is a brief convulsive spell. Gastaut (1974) described the muscular events of the convulsive syncope as tonic spasms. Others have reported that true clonic movements do not occur with syncope, but only sudden tonic postures (Duvoisin, 1962; Ferris et al., 1934). Careful observation of syncopal spells shows that clonic flexion movements, or at least briefly repetitive twitching, are not uncommon. In a retrospective study of syncopal blood donors, Ziegler et al. (1978) found reports of some convulsive movements in one seventh. In a prospective study they found 106 blood donors had syncope without movements but 65 had some form of movement during the spell. They emphasized, however, that none of their subjects had the characteristic tonic-clonic sequence typical of generalized cerebral seizures.

Convulsive movements or tonic spasms which are a result of syncope can be distinguished from epileptic seizures by three characteristics: 1) they begin with a syncopal slump; 2) they lack a typical tonic-clonic sequence; and 3) they have a very brief postictal phase. A setting or history conducive to syncope is also suggestive (Edmondson, 1978). When these key features are overlooked in the face of "jerking movements" with dramatic occurrence of a sudden loss of consciousness, the diagnosis of epileptic seizures may be made even before syncope is considered.

PATHOPHYSIOLOGY AND ETIOLOGY OF SYNCOPE

The final common mechanism in all forms of syncope is hypoxic interruption of brain function (Gastaut, 1974). Several different mechanisms may cause such interruption (see Table 3.1). The clinical phase of lipothymia, or presyncope, is marked by diffuse 3–5 Hz slow waves on EEG which occurs within 2 seconds after a drop in pulse rate or blood pressure (Engel et al, 1944; Gestaut and Fischer-Williams, 1957). Loss of consciousness and postural tone are heralded by slower, rhythmical delta waves (1–3 Hz) on EEG if bradycardia or hypotension persists. This same sequence occurs in syncope due to any mechanism. When compression or other maneuvers capable of causing syncope are performed as the subject breathes 100% oxygen, the characteristic sequence of lipothymia, progression of EEG changes, and complete loss of consciousness may be slowed or averted. As soon as the pulse or blood pressure is restored and the subject is made recumbent or supine, EEG patterns return to normal and the subject quickly awakens. In syncope, during the period of unconsciousness, eye movements, pupillary responses, and brain stem evoked responses remain normal. This supports

Table 3.1
Syncope

I. Reflex Syncopes—Vasovagal or Vasodepressor Syncope
   A. Carotid sinus syndrome
   B. Psychogenic or neurogenic fainting (may be different from "hysterical" fainting)
   C. Micturition syncope
   D. Tussive syncope
   E. Valsalva-maneuver syncope
II. Syncope due to Cardiac Causes
   A. Irregularities of rhythm
      1. Heart block with Adams-Stokes syndrome
      2. Supraventricular arrhythmias; sinoatrial block; atrial fibrillation, paroxysmal atrial tachycardia, "sick sinus syndrome"
      3. Frequent ventricular premature beats
   B. Failure to compensate for sudden drops in peripheral vascular resistance
      1. Congenital heart disease (shunts)
      2. Myxoma
      3. Ball-valve thrombus
      4. Mitral valve disease or prolapse
      5. Myocardial diseases (myocarditis, degenerative diseases, ischemia)
III. Syncope due to (Noncardiac) Perfusion Failure
   A. Orthostatic hypotension
      1. Hypovolemia
      2. Primary central dysautonomia, CNS degenerative disease (Parkinson's disease)
      3. Autonomic peripheral neuropathy
      4. Medications (mostly antihypertensives)
   B. Shock—may not require postural changes
   C. Cerebrovascular disease
IV. Syncope due to Anoxia
V. Syncope with Convulsive Movements (Convulsive Syncope)

the concept that cerebral hypoxia or hypoperfusion accounts for the clinical features. Although there have been isolated reports of epileptiform sharp waves in some syncope (Lloyd-Smith and Tatlow, 1953), the slow wave patterns described above are virtually universal. When hypoperfusion persists, EEG slow waves are followed by diffuse voltage supression ("flattening") of the EEG trace (Gastaut and Fischer-Williams, 1957; Gastaut and Gastaut, 1958; Engel, 1963). This sequence of EEG slowing followed by voltage suppresion can also be produced by experimental or operative impairments of cerebral perfusion or oxygenation. Because convulsive movements when present in syncope occur only after "flattening" of EEG activity, Gastaut concluded that the movements are due to loss of cortical inhibition and release of bulbo-pontine postural reflexes (Gastaut and Gastaut, 1958; Gastaut, 1974). These movements are usually brief, often only one extensor spasm, and they seem to represent a surrender of cortical function, specifically the loss of cortical inhibition releasing brain stem reflexes, as do other features of syncope. In the presence of preexisting cerebral disease or regional vascular deficits, cerebral hypotension may induce focal convulsions which incriminate local cortical mechanisms (Riley and Friedman, 1981); however, preservation of consciousness and other clinical features suggest this phenomenon is not truly a part of the syncope spectrum.

REFLEX SYNCOPE

The most common forms of syncope, and least likely to be associated with other medical complaints, are those due to the "syncopal reflex" (Gastaut, 1974; Engel, 1962 and 1978; Brick, 1978). In all forms of the reflex syncopes, an autonomic outflow traceable to pontine and medullary structures leads to peripheral blood pooling, diminished cardiac output, or both. Braunwald (1980) emphasized the role of the carotid sinus baroreceptor reflex in cardiac function. He distinguished the reflex syncopes due to carotid sinus reflex, which have prominent cardioinhibitory features, from the pure vasodepressor syncopes, which may be due to sudden arterial hypotension without any change in pulse rate or cardiac output.

The reflex syncopes are not confined only to what Gastaut calls "emotive" syncopes. A hypersensitivity to vagal tone through the vasodepressor reflex (demonstrated by Gastaut) may cause syncope with compression of the carotid sinus, urination, coughing, or the Valsalva maneuver. The general sensitivity to the vasodepressor syndrome tends to have a familial clustering in incidence, and even the particular triggers may be common among family members. This is particularly true in micturition-induced syncope in which males, perhaps because they urinate standing and thus are more vulnerable to diminished cardiac return, are affected more often than females.

The baroreceptors in the carotid sinus are among the most important for gauging and regulating blood pressure The nerve of Hering from the carotid sinus joins the glossopharyngeal nerve and enters the brain stem to synapse in the nucleus tractus solitarius, dorsal motor nucleus of the vagus, and the medullary reticular formation. Pressure elevation within the carotid sinus is normally followed with an almost immediate response from the neurons in the dorsal motor nucleus of the vagus with slowing of the pulse, with delay of sinoatrial transmission, and often with diminished cardiac output. Under most circumstances, directly increasing pressure in the carotid sinus without influencing other baroreceptors elicits a reflex response confined to vagus and cardiac functions, apparently entirely mediated by acetylcholine. Diseases which affect either the glossopharyngeal nerve, carotid sinus, or cardiac sensitivity to acetylcholine may render subjects vulnerable to what ordinarily would be trivial activation of carotid sinus reflex. There are also subjects who seem to have an idiopathic hypersensitivity to stimulation of the carotid sinus. Predisposing conditions include atherosclerosis involving the carotid sinus and autonomic peripheral neuropathies, particularly those due to diabetes (Ewing et al, 1980). Pressure over the region of the carotid bifurcation, simple turning of the neck, shaving, or wearing tight collars may lead to activation of the carotid sinus and subsequent cardioinhibitory responses and frank asystole, leading to syncope and, rarely, to death (Engel, 1978; Braunwald, 1980; Davies et al., 1979).

Other afferent impulses from the glossopharyngeal nerve may lead to activation of the vagal cardioinhibitory reflex, leading to syncope. These include oropharyngeal pain, or idiopathic inflammation and pain syndromes of the glossopharyngeal nerve (Taylor, 1977). Other forms of sudden sensory stimulation of cranial nerves which may lead to profound bradycardia or cardiac arrest through vagal mediated mechanisms include sudden cold stimulation (as with cold wind or water) (Brick, 1978), eye pain, and sudden head or neck movements.

Vasodepressor Reflexes

In other forms of reflex syncope there may be no evidence of direct cardiac inhibition but only a sudden drop in peripheral vascular tone leading to profound hypotension, diminished cardiac output and, hence, syncope. Three major types of stimuli seem capable of triggering the vasodepressor syncopal reflex: psychological, corneopalpebral sensation, and visceral sensory inputs (Gastaut, 1974; Engel, 1962, 1978). Usually, vagal outflow (cholinergic mechanisms) and sympathetic vascular effects (epinephrine mediated) occur together. Although vagotomy or anticholinergic drugs may avert bradycardia or arrhythmia, reflex vasodepressor mechanisms causing diminished peripheral vascular resistance and venous pooling remain. Profound arterial vasodilation in skeletal muscle, presumed by Engel to be an expression of preparation for "flight or fight" response, may alone be sufficient to cause syncope.

The vasodepressor reflex may be initiated by intracardiac receptors in response to increased ventricular pressures or volumes, whether due to outflow obstruction, heart block, or arrhythmia (Aviado and Schmidt, 1959). Such a mechanism may operate in micturition-induced syncope, because anticholinergic medications which counteract cardioinhibitory functions may also avert vasodepressor features. Fatigue, prior alcohol consumption, and sleep interruption (all of which may aggravate medullary-cardiac reflexes) exacerbate micturition-related syncope. Symptoms often begin around puberty and seem to continue throughout adulthood, often growing worse in late middle age coincident with prostatic hypertrophy and greater abdominal and parasympathetic efforts at urination.

The most common form of syncope is the sudden vagal/vasodepressor reflex triggered by emotional stress called "common faint" by Braunwald (1980). The terms "neurogenic" and "psychogenic" suggest the useful concepts of a neural reflex and psychological base to the sequence. The mere viewing of an object with emotional symbolism may excite the reflex in susceptible people. This differs from other forms of reflex syncope in that the precipitant is not a primary vascular or humoral perturbation such as Valsalva maneuver or cholinergic outflow. Psychogenic vasodepressor syncope should also be distinguished from the ordinary concept of "hysterical syncope," which refers to swooning without change in pulse or blood pressure. Psychogenic syncope is a direct physiological disorder, albeit in response to a fundamentally psychological trigger; the hysterical faint or malingered faint occurs without physiological substrate.

A curiosity in psychogenic syncope is that loss of consciousness often is more rapid than expected if anoxia of cerebral structures alone accounted for the episode. Perhaps consciousness is lost more slowly than an observer perceives, and a period of retrograde amnesia after a spell may prevent recall of premonitory symptoms. Alternately ascending inhibitory impulses linked with autonomic reflexes may cause almost instantaneous arrests of consciousness by reticular formation inhibition, as in some forms of cataplexy.

Little is known about the precise anatomy of the afferent pathways responsible for psychogenic syncope. The striking biphasic quality of cardiovascular phenomena begins with increase in heart rate, in total systemic resistance, and in blood pressure, when the patient may appear apprehensive but not acknowledge it. Suddenly, atrial pressure, cardiac output, pulse rate, peripheral vascular resistance, and blood pressure all drop. Engel and Romano (1947) interpreted the initial phase as a sympathetic preparedness for flight or fight, but they interpreted the second vasodepressor phase as a physiologic confusion between a continued preparedness state (increased muscle blood flow and diminished peripheral vascular resistance) and a paradoxical inclination to lie down and withdraw or conserve energy (bradycardia and diminished cardiac output). Engel suggested that syncope represents a "failure of mechanisms that normally maintain linkage between cardiovascular processes and somatic needs." The "crucial psychological variable is the degree of unresolvable uncertainty" presented by a particular circumstance, and syncope may be analogous to sham death used by some animals as a means of avoiding unwinnable conflict (Romano and Engel, 1945).

The paradigm is the apprehensive individual who feels confronted with an insurmountable threat and no apparent acceptable escape who also feels a need to maintain a facade or appearance of mastery. There are many instances of cardiac death under such circumstances, even among subjects without preexisting cardiac disease (Engel, 1978).

SYNCOPE DUE TO NONCARDIAC PERFUSION FAILURE

Postural change from supine or sitting posture to an upright position must be accompanied by an instantaneous increase in vasomotor tone and venous return in order to maintain normal blood pressure and cardiac return. Occasional hypotensive spells commonly cause sensations of lipothymia in normal people who rise rapidly from bed or chair. Failure of autonomic vasotonic reflexes necessary to maintain pressure and pulse rate may result from central mechanisms, as occur in familial central dysautonomia, Shy-Drager syndrome, and Parkinson's disease. In peripheral neuropathies which particularly affect autonomic nerves—such as diabetes, porphyria or amyloid—syncope may be a significant cause of disability (Watkins and McKay, 1980; Ewing et al., 1980). Medications may block peripheral vasomotor tone (tricyclic antidepressants, phenothiazines, dopa, hydralazine) or postganglionic sympathetic transmission (guanethidine). A clear-cut relationship of spells to postural changes, e.g., recurrent lipothymia upon standing and rapid recovery on becoming recumbent, should make the diagnosis obvious. However, many subjects susceptible to this condition have postictal amnesia for the initial events and, therefore, many complain only of the fall. If actual epileptic seizures are strongly suggested by history, electroencephalography should be a part of the evaluation (Riley and Friedman, 1981).

Distinguishing between micturition syncope and orthostatic hypotension may be difficult among older men who arise at night to urinate (Gastaut and Gastaut, 1958; Donker et al., 1972) but can usually be resolved by measuring blood pressure and pulse before and after rising from the supine position, by the history of recent onset of symptoms (micturition syncope often begins in younger men or may be present for many years) and by the fact that the symptoms or fainting spells occur immediately before or during urination. Orthostatic hypotension may not induce complete collapse until the cardiac output falls several minutes after the subject arises from bed, thus allowing him to walk into an adjacent room. In persons prone to micturition syncope, the mere anticipation of voiding is sufficient to induce an attack.

Gastaut has described exertion syncopes which seem to occur entirely among older people and which seem to be caused by vasovagal maneuvers, coughing, or laryngeal stress during marked physical effort. Such exertional syncopes are probably examples of the hyperactive carotid sinus syndrome.

CARDIAC CAUSES

Syncope with complete heartblock, the so-called Stokes-Adams syndrome, is commonly presumed to be the most common cause of cardiac-related syncope. However, the mechanism responsible for syncope, even among patients with complete heart block is most often a ventricular arrhythmia superimposed at the time that consciousness is lost, rather than the heart block *per se* (Pomerantz and O'Rourke, 1969). So the term "arrhythmia-induced syncope" may be more accurate (Braunwald, 1980). Fifty thousand new cases of heart block occur annually in the United States, and 50% of these patients have at least one syncopal spell (Braunwald, 1980).

The different types of arrhythmias and mechanisms capable of inducing syncope fall into five major classes:

1. Transitory, complete interruption of atrioventricular conduction with asystole during a "pre-automatic pause" or "warm-up" interval, before a supraventricular pacemaker can supervene.
2. Asystole, in the presence of perisistent complete heart block due to failure of an intranodal pacemaker.
3. Paroxysmal ventricular tachycardia or fibrillation which may be precipitated by ischemia due to slow heart rate with complete block or due to overdrive suppression of an ectopic ventricular focus.
4. Supraventricular tachycardia or bradyarrhythmias leading to poor cardiac output. Ischemia may result from such mechanisms and secondarily lead to ventricular tachycardia.
5. Combinations of conduction disturbances and supraventricular arrhythmias, often associated with the "sick sinus syndrome."

Aside from arrhythmias, cardiac disease or dysfunction may cause cerebral hypoperfusion because of diminished contractibility or outflow obstruction. This is usually not due to a drop in cardiac output but rather a failure to *increase* output in face of greater demand. The failure to increase output with postural change or during vigorous exertion, when increased blood flow to muscle causes a drop in peripheral vascular resistance, is responsible for the characteristic feature of syncope on exertion. Systemic vascular resistance ordinarily declines as a consequence of arteriolar dilatation secondary to the accumulation of metabolites such as carbon dioxide and lactate during exercise. Normally, vasodilation is more than compensated by the augmentation of cardiac output during exertion. In diseases in which output cannot rise proportionately to the fall in vascular resistance, the resultant drop in blood pressure leads to impaired cerebral perfusion and, ultimately, syncope.

Outflow obstruction or valvular lesions are the most common impediments to cardiac output which lead to syncope. Paradoxically, the increased ventricular or atrial pressures due to ventricular outflow obstruction may activate both cardiac baroreceptors and vasodepressor reflexes. Although these reflexes attempt to compensate for end-diastolic cardiac pressures, they in turn further depress vascular resistances; this leads to syncope. Pedunculated masses, such as atrial myxomata or ball-valve thrombi, may obstruct outflow only when particular postures are assumed and, thus, cause syncope sporadically—particularly when there are changes in posture.

Lesions extrinsic to the heart may also cause hypotension by outflow obstruction or by inducing secondary arrhythmias. These include pulmonary embolus, obstruction of the aorta due to Takayasu's disease or coarctation, and tamponade of the heart, such as pericardial effusion or hemorrhage.

DIFFERENTIAL DIAGNOSIS: "FIT VS. FAINT"

To emphasize the difficulty in distinguishing epilepsy and syncope and the magnitude of this problem, it is worthwhile to consider the number of patients who carry an initial diagnosis of epilepsy but are eventually found to have syncope. Gastaut and Gastaut (1958) reported 946 subjects referred for intensive study of episodic loss of consciousness. Of 265 patients referred by neuropsychiatrists or pediatricians, 252 had an original diagnosis of epilepsy; only 3 came with a diagnosis of syncope. Another 681 were referred by general practitioners: with the diagnosis of epilepsy in 309 cases, syncope in 111 cases, and unknown etiology in 261 cases. After intensive monitoring and diagnostic procedures utilizing activation EEG and polygraphic recording, syncope was diagnosed in 417 cases (44%) and was 10% more common than epilepsy—the final diagnosis for 377 subjects. After complete evaluation, the number of diagnoses of epilepsy was reduced by 30%. Schott et al. (1979) found that 20% of patients referred for epilepsy actually had chronic cardiac arrhythmia (sinoatrial arrhythmia was particularly common). They noted that neurological dysfunction is frequently a manifestation of cardiac disease, exemplified by one elderly patient whose initial complaint was episodic confusional spells. When his cardiac arrhythmia was treated, episodic confusion improved.

Others have shown that dizziness and falling may be particularly common in elderly patients with chronic mental disease and may lead to inappropriate treatment with antiepileptic drugs. In one series, 40% of elderly demented patients complained of episodic dizziness and falling, and 25% of these had demonstrable orthostatic hypotension and syncope (Blumenthal and Davie, 1980). The "sick sinus syndrome" is a form of coronary sinus pacemaker instability which causes episodic bradyarrhythmia and frequent junctional or ventricular premature beats and frequently causes episodic neurological dysfunction and syncope (Sutton and Perrins, 1977). Among patients with transient neurologic deficits, as many as one third have hemodynamically significant cardiac rhythm abnormalities when studied by 24-hour electrocardiographic monitoring, but only 3% of age- and sex-matched individuals without neurologic symptoms show such abnormalities.

The physical examination of the person with possible syncope or seizures must include, in addition to neurologic and cardiac examinations, blood pressure recording in both arms and legs, blood pressure recumbent and standing for at least 3 minutes, auscultation for cervical and abdominal bruits, and examination of extremities for signs of congenital heart disease, such as clubbing or cyanosis.

One basic tenet of physiologic recording for evaluation of episodic loss of consciousness is to record all potentially important functions during one of the patient's typical spells. Cardiac monitors are routinely used in most modern EEG laboratories, and many laboratories include respiratory monitors, transducers to record body movement, and videotape monitoring for special cases. Just as it is important to include the appropriate stimulus in recording the EEG of an individual who may have reflex epilepsy, it is likewise important to undertake appropriate maneuvers to induce and record a typical spell in a person who may have micturition—or orthostatic—syncope. Since syncope is usually accompanied by high voltage slow waves on EEG and may even be accompanied by sharp waves (Lloyd-Smith and Tatlow, 1953), it may be important to have constant blood pressure monitoring as well as EKG monitoring to accompany EEG in a person for whom the distinction is particularly difficult.

As intensive monitoring and long-term recording techniques have revolutionized the study of epileptic seizures, portable EKG recorders which can be used during normal activity demonstrate many cardiac conduction abnormalities not seen on conventional cardiac examinations. In one study, 32% of patients with transient neurologic symptoms had hemodynamically significant conduction abnormalities when studied by long-term EKG monitoring; 12 of 60 such subjects had been previously considered to have epileptic seizures, while 70% of those who had hemodynamically significant abnormalities had two or more distinct types of abnormalities, including atrioventricular dissociation, ectopic ventricular beats, and ectopic atrial beats (Luxon et al., 1980).

Laboratory assessments include serum electrolytes, catecholamines both in the supine and upright positions, dopamine β-hydroxylase, and urinary vanillyl mandelic acid (VMA). Under physiologic conditions, catecholamines increase several fold with upright posture, but with idiopathic orthostatic hypotension or autonomic neuropathy there may be no change. In such patients, plasma dopamine β-hydroxylase levels may also be low and fail to rise with postural change. Although pheochromocytomas usually secrete norepinephrine, they sometimes secrete epinephrine, eliciting an unexpected episodic hypotension. Glucose tolerance tests may be useful, particularly with simultaneous insulin assays, although hypoglycemia is suspected much more often than it is found to cause symptoms.

SUMMARY

Generalized tonic-clonic seizures begin with a tonic phase, which may be unilateral. Subsequently a slow clonic type of movement may begin focally and then become bilateral and synchronous. A generalized tonic or tonic-clonic seizure seldom begins with a slow slumping collapse and even less often begins with a feeling of gradual blurring of consciousness. Premonitory symptoms may be focal sensory abnormalities, bizarre affective premonitions, or hallucinations but are seldom a mere "light headedness." Likewise, irregular pulse or dramatic fall in blood pressure, particularly if associated with postural changes, is often seen with syncope but is seldom seen with seizures. An exception is the "temporal lobe syncope" described by Caffi (1973) and Delgado-Escueta (1979). Probably the most important observation is the distinction between the flaccidity or swooning at the onset of an attack which typifies most syncopal spells and the rigidity, stiffness, or bizarre mental symptoms which typify epileptic seizures.

TREATMENT OF SYNCOPE

Treatment of syncope ultimately depends upon treating the underlying *cause* and is seldom satisfying. Ironically, because an underlying mechanism can be identified and dealt with, hysterical swooning may be more treatable than other causes of blackouts. Pacemakers or medical therapy may be more effective for syncope due to cardiac arrhythmias, and surgery is often necessary to correct cardiac or arterial outflow lesions. Recurrent syncope due to central or peripheral autonomic failure or to reflex syncope mechanisms is more resistant. Blocking vagal outflow with anticholinergic medications is often effective, as may be vagotomy for carefully selected patients or section of Hering's nerve for carotid sinus sensitivity. Unfortunately, however, vagal interruption may only affect reflex cardiac functions, bradycardia or heart block. As important as these phenomena may be, the peripheral vasodepressor response, primarily an adrenergic mechanism, may still cause syncope or disabling lipothymia. Artificial mineralocorticoids, usually fluorinated compounds (fluorocortisone or fluoroprednisolone) may increase fluid volume and compensate for syncope associated with adrenal insufficiency; to some degree, such volume expansion may be helpful also for patients with autonomic failure (Shy-Drager syndrome or Parkinson's disease). Antigravity stockings to the waist or midtorso are useful in some patients, but in order to significantly affect venous return they must be so tight that they are usually very uncomfortable and may be impossible for elderly or movement-impaired individuals to put on by themselves. As venous pooling is usually not the major influence in syncopal hypertension and antigravity stockings do not affect arterial or arteriolar capacitance, they offer only partial relief to many patients.

Often, to merely recognize syncope and distinguish it from epilepsy is sufficient treatment. As antiepileptic drugs are often administered, an appropriate diagnosis may eliminate the use of harmful medication which may include hypotensive or autonomic side effects.

Hyperventilation

First described as "sighing dyspnea" in 1929 by White and Hahn, the acute attack of hyperventilation in response to stress has since been frequently described. The most familiar and easily recognizable pattern occurs in the adolescent or young adult. He or she complains of an inability to breathe deeply enough (despite appearance to the contrary), complains of acroparesthesia, and has carpopedal spasm—or even frank tetany (Ames, 1955; Engel et al., 1947; Pincus, 1970). There is usually a precipitating emotional stress (Engel, 1968; Lum, 1975). Symptoms are promptly resolved by having the patient rebreathe expired air from a paper bag placed over the nose and mouth.

While hyperventilation has frequently been described, the diversity

Table 3.2
Most Common Manifestations of Hyperventilation Syndrome

Neurological
  1. Central: Dizziness, sense of unreality, loss of consciousness, blurred vision,
        anxiety
  2. Peripheral: Paresthesiae, tetany, muscle spasm
Cardiovascular: Palpitations, tachycardia, precardiac pain, Raynaud's phenom-
        enon
Respiratory: Shortness of breath, chest pain, "asthma"
Gastrointestinal: Heartburn, aerophagia, epigastric pain, nausea gilobus
Musculoskeletal: Muscle cramps, weakness, easy fatigability

and subtlety of the clinical manifestations are not very frequently
recognized (Table 3.2). Lum (1975) called the classical, obvious cases
"tip of the iceberg," because the bulk of cases either go unrecognized or
are mistaken for other conditions—frequently epilepsy. In one series of
128 patients with nonorganic complaints leading to a medical evaluation,
21 patients had twitching eyelids, headache, giddiness, or fainting as
the condition which most frequently led to confusion resulting in a
diagnosis of neurologic disease. Another 16 patients had episodic weakness or vague pains. The possibility of seizures had been entertained in
diagnosing both groups (Gottlieb, 1969). Tetany induced by hyperventilation causes spasm or shaking in extremities and is often sudden in
onset and may appear epileptic (Engel et al., 1947; Fraser and Sargent,
1929; Ames, 1955; Stead and Warren, 1943). Other symptoms which
mimic seizures may be focal paresthesias, feelings of "insects crawling,"
dizziness, blurring of vision, and feelings of unreality (Engel, 1968; Lum,
1975; Stead and Warren, 1943; Pincus, 1978). Such symptoms, particularly if followed by loss of consciousness or motor manifestations, may
suggest "auras" of complex partial seizures. The preceding hyperventilation may not be recognized as the primary pathologic process but may
erroneously be interpreted as a mere precipitant of an epileptic seizure.

The hyperventilation syndrome is more common than is recognized.
Pincus (1978) found adequate information for the diagnosis in 30 of 550
patients in a neurology clinic over a 5-year period. Pfeffer (1978) reported that in 6–11% of patients seen in a general medical practice, a
major portion of symptoms were directly attributable to involuntary
hyperventilation. In a 10-year period, Lum (1975) found 700 patients
with the hyperventilation syndrome who had no detectable pathological
state related to respiration functions, but he excluded a large number of
patients in whom cardiopulmonary disease might have affected analysis
of the data. He concluded that the *recognized* number of people with
the hyperventilation *syndrome* represents the minority of people with

hyperventilation-induced symptoms. The patients with unrecognized hyperventilation often have bizarre symptoms affecting different organ systems. Lum points out that many such patients have the "multiple doctor" or "fat folder" syndrome. Burns and Howell (1969) found that 10% of patients complaining of dyspnea in a cardiologic practice had episodic hyperventilation due to anxiety. In another study, 40% of patients in a medical outpatient clinic had no detectable organic disease but did have symptoms suggesting hyperventilation (Goettlieb, 1969).

DIAGNOSTIC DIFFICULTY

Given the prevalence of the condition and the pathophysiology attributable to overbreathing, it may be surprising that the correct diagnosis can be overlooked. Patients seldom complain of overbreathing per se (Engel et al., 1947; Kerr et al., 1937), and the common impression that hyperventilation attacks are only sudden dramatic episodes of gasping and tetany may be misleading (Lewis, 1953, 1954). It is true that in most series of *reported* and hence *recognized* cases of the syndrome, cardio-pulmonary complaints or diagnosis outnumbered suspected neurologic disease, but 80% of subjects have some alterations of consciousness during attacks (Pincus, 1978) and, in most series, 20% of subjects have been labeled epileptic or syncopal, or they have been subjected to diagnostic procedures because of suspected epilepsy (Joorabchi, 1977; Lum, 1975). In fact, 6–15% of patients lose consciousness during hyperventilation attacks (Ames, 1955; Pincus, 1978). Fraser and Sargant (1938) reported that 20 consecutive patients referred for "fits" actually suffered from hyperventilation attacks, not epilepsy. Although tetany and paresthesia usually occur in a distal and symmetrical manner, such symptoms may be asymmetrical or affect only one extremity (Kerr et al., 1937; Lewis, 1953). When the individual complains of gradual blurring of consciousness, followed by "blackout" and accompanied or heralded by unilateral paresthesia, focal epileptic seizures may seem likely.

ILLUSTRATIVE CASES

Case 1. A 24-year-old woman with a long history of "grand mal seizures" was referred for her fifth neurologic evaluation because of uncontrolled seizures. Her initial "seizure" at age 16 did *not* cause complete loss of consciousness but left her weak and sleepy for half an hour. Although she and her parents could not recall the exact details of that episode, they were told by the neurologist that it was a grand mal seizure. An EEG obtained shortly afterward reportedly showed high voltage sharp and slow waves "of an atypical spike wave pattern during hyperventilation." She was subsequently treated with varying doses of primidone, phenytoin, ethosuximide and, most recently, valproic acid. The initial EEG was reviewed and found to be normal, showing only a normal degree of high voltage slow activity induced by hyperventilation. Her parents reported that her right arm grew rigid at the onset of spells, and that she would warn of an impending spell. In some spells she fell and became rigid, with wrists and hands flexed and turned outward. She sometimes slept after the spells, but most often her mother noted that she was irritable, diaphoretic, and seemed perhaps to breathe more deeply.

Several EEGs, including an all-night sleep recording, were normal. When she was asked to overbreathe, the EEG had diffuse high voltage slow waves, but she did not complain of typical symptoms. Simultaneous closed-circuit television and EEG telemetry clearly showed that rapid deep breathing and high voltage slow waves on EEG occurred together during her typical spells. When overbreathing and slow waves were seen on telemetry monitors, she was asked to rebreathe in a paper bag and her symptoms remitted completely.

Case 2. A 24-year-old sailor had recurrent feelings of unreality and distance from the environment, occasionally followed by generalized tonic postures and unconsciousness. When these spells began, his shipmates noted a gradual "change in personality." His neurologic examination and EEG were normal, but when he hyperventilated he became rigid and the EEG was obscured by head movement and muscle artifact. The original EEG reported that a "grand mal seizure" had been triggered by hyperventilation, and treatment with phenytoin was initiated. The spells recurred and, as higher doses of phenytoin failed to control them, the patient was referred to a larger center.

During the spontaneous spells, it was noted that he had sternal anterior chest excursion breathing and no abdominal excursions and that whenever he breathed into a paper bag the spells could be aborted immediately. Abnormalities were never recorded on the EEG. Subsequently, it was learned that he was anxious and afraid on the ship, and his "personality change," initially attributed to temporal lobe changes, was found to be due to depression.

Case 3. A 16-year-old girl with a history of absence seizures had been seizure-free for 5 years with ethosuximide "treatment." Two months before neurologic referral, her doctor had added valproic acid because she had begun to have "recurrence of seizures." Previous seizures had been momentary staring spells with no movements. Her new spells consisted of rigidity of the upper extremities, blurring of consciousness, and generalized shaking movements. They often began with focal tingling and stiffening of the left arm.

When her seizures were first recognized, she was particularly sensitive to overbreathing which induced vigorous high voltage spike and wave patterns on EEG and quickly triggered absence seizures. A recent EEG had been completely normal, as she was still receiving ethosuximide. With vigorous hyperventilation for 5 minutes, she began to complain of tingling in her left arm and then of flexor spasms of both upper extremities. She became visibly anxious and complained that she was "about to have a spell." She did not lose consciousness completely but ceased speaking. Her eyelids fluttered rapidly as both upper extremities began to tremble and her legs were extended. The EEG showed high voltage irregular 3 per second slow waves with a "notch" contour but no spike and wave discharges. After she stopped hyperventilating, the carpopedal spasm continued for 2 minutes until the slow waves disappeared from the EEG. After 30 minutes the overbreathing was repeated, and when she began to complain of tingling in one arm she was offered a bag for rebreathing. Within 30 seconds the EEG changed and symptoms disappeared completely. Later, overbreathing was repeated with the patient breathing 100% oxygen. The EEG remained normal; she did not stop speaking; however, spasms in her hands and feet still occurred.

She had a clear history of epilepsy, and medication had controlled her absence seizures. The new spells were quite different from her previous seizures, but she was at a typical age for the evolution of generalized tonic-clonic seizures in a person with childhood absence spells. This case illustrates the importance of a high index of suspicion for hyperventilation syndrome and once again emphasizes the importance of recognizing that episodic spells of other etiology may coexist with epileptic seizures. Engel et al. (1947) noted that hyperventilation seldom triggers generalized tonic-clonic or partial seizures.

PHYSIOLOGIC BASIS OF SYMPTOMS

The clinical features of hyperventilation and hypocapnia fall into three major categories: peripheral neuromuscular manifestations (paresthesia, muscle cramps and tetany); cerebral or "central" neurologic manifestations (sense of unreality, sense of impending loss of consciousness, light-headedness, frank loss of consciousness); and autonomic manifestations (tachycardia, peripheral vasoconstriction, increased peripheral vascular resistance, and palpitations). Although the pathophysiological substrate of the cerebral manifestations is now clearly attributable to diminished brain oxygen tension, the peripheral manifestations are apparently due to altered arterial concentration of ionized calcium, which (unlike cerebral symptoms) are not paralleled by EEG changes. Some have suggested that central (CNS) symptoms and peripheral manifestations seldom coincide (Engel et al., 1947), although most series show a significant coincidence of both central and peripheral manifestations. In many individuals the accompanying autonomic manifestations precede the onset of other clinical features. The autonomic manifestations may be a product of the same stress precipitant which leads to the hyperventilation attack. It has been demonstrated that the mere act of hyperventilation in volunteers may lead to peripheral vasoconstriction, tachycardia, and hypertension. Perhaps the act of overbreathing may precipitate autonomic features without causing other cerebral symptoms (Ames, 1955).

Haldane and Poulton (1908) reported paresthesia and pain with voluntary hyperventilation as well as a "peculiar sense of giddiness" which they suggested resembled anoxia. Their earliest interpretations of the sensory and mental changes due to hyperventilation were that the diminished arterial pCO_2 suppressed neuronal excitability. Henderson (1909) noted that after hyperventilation performed passively on anesthesized dogs there was usually a prolonged apnea. Ames (1955) noted that subjects with involuntary spells of subconscious hyperventilation usually did not exhibit this posthyperventilation apnea. Hill and Flack (1910) first mentioned vascular effects of overbreathing, reporting diminished pulse amplitude and decreased systolic blood pressure. The first comparison of overbreathing to tetany was made by Grant and Goldman in 1920. They subsequently demonstrated that the serum calcium levels in their subjects were normal despite recorded arterial alkalosis. Although they were unable to measure ionized calcium fractions, they correctly concluded that "a portion of the calcium is in some way rendered inactive though still present in the circulating blood" (1920).

Goldman (1922) observed 11 subjects who had sudden spasms or tetanic postures from hyperventilation, and two persons with hysterical pseudotetany, and pointed out that "some cases of hysterical pseudotetany are undoubtedly . . . due to over-respiration." He did not, however, associate the involuntary overbreathing with emotional stress, although he did observe that the syndrome of involuntary overbreathing was a recurrent pattern in many individuals.

Rosett (1924) noted that voluntary overbreathing could uncover neurological deficits and thought that hyperventilation caused exaggerated neuronal function. Since 1940 when Gibbs et al. demonstrated that hyperventilation could precipitate both absence seizures and the characteristic spike and wave EEG pattern, this procedure became a standard feature of routine EEG recording. Davis and Wallace (1942) demonstrated that many apparently normal individuals had very prominent high voltage delta waves induced on EEG following hyperventilation and that there was a consistent rise in arterial pH which paralleled the drop in arterial pCO_2. All subsequent investigators found that giddiness, light-headedness, anxiety, and other mental status changes always correlated with the eruption of high voltage delta waves on EEG (Stead and Warren, 1943; Engel, et al., 1947). Kety and Schmidt (1946) demonstrated that systemic and cerebral vascular resistance increased with hyperventilation. Breathing 100% oxygen or administering vasodilators was shown to prevent cerebral symptoms of hyperventilation, but calcium infusions did not (Engel et al., 1947; Davis and Wallace, 1940). These studies led to the conclusion that hyperventilation-induced hypocapnea leads to systemic and cerebral vasoconstriction and, hence, diminished cerebral blood flow and diminished cerebral oxygenation (Gotoh et al., 1965; Raichle et al., 1972; Kennealy et al., 1980; Adams and Severinghaus, 1962).

Reivich (1964) showed that diminished arterial pCO_2 did indeed diminish total cerebral blood flow and further showed that this effect was due to increased cerebral vascular resistance (CVR). Since arterial pCO_2 often does not correlate with cerebral blood flow, Lassen (1968) concluded that alteration of extracellular brain pH was responsible for cerebral vascular response to hyperventilation. In Lassen's view, interstitial fluid pH was the major mechanism of CO_2 influence on cerebral blood flow. Plum and Posner (1972) attributed the effects of prolonged hyperventilation to accumulation of lactic acid. Whatever the mechanism, it is clear that hyperventilation can significantly decrease the total cerebral blood flow as much as 30–40% (Raichle et al., 1970; Gotoh et al., 1965; Kennealy et al., 1980; Raichle and Plum, 1972).

ETIOLOGY OF HYPERVENTILATION ATTACKS

There may be several reasons for recurring attacks of involuntary or unconscious overbreathing. Pfeffer (1978) and Lowry (1967) first noted that there are several different dynamic mechanisms which may predispose to overbreathing, either during stress or merely in anticipation of it. Burns and Howell (1969) found the respiratory rate to be higher among depressed patients than among controls, with a correlation between respiratory rate and severity of depression. Not only is respiration faster and deeper among depressed patients than among controls (Damas Mora et al., 1976) but also depression scales are elevated in at least 40% of subjects with the hyperventilation syndrome (Pfeffer, 1978). Depression may, therefore, be a significant underlying factor in the disorder. It is likely that depression is the major feature of the *chronic hyperventilation syndrome* discussed below. Subjects with chronic, subclinical degrees of overbreathing who do not manifest tetany or noticeable cerebral symptoms may nonetheless be more vulnerable to mild changes in respiratory rate because of chronic hypocapnia and a diminished "hyperventilatory reserve." Lowry (1967) found that hyperventilators among military recruits regarded themselves as physically inferior, had family histories of cardiothoracic illness, and were preoccupied with body functions. Others have noted that childhood histories of emotional instability, family history of neurosis, and failure of psychosexual adjustment are prevalent among such patients (Glieb and Auerbach, 1944). Such a background predisposes to attacks of over-breathing when faced with conflict, threatening indecision, or intolerable stress. Lowry (1967) and Pfeffer (1978) suggested that hyperventilation may represent an avoidance mechanism for coping with stress.

Since increased ventilatory volume and rate occur too rapidly to be compensatory for exercise, deep and rapid breathing may be viewed simply as preparation for the "flight or fight" response (Engel, 1968; Pfeffer, 1978; Ames, 1955; Lewis, 1954). Lazarus and Kostan (1969) suggest that hyperventilators typically are "running scared" and are often obsessed with fear, e.g., of death, of developing a fatal illness, of losing their minds, or of loneliness. Such constant anxiety and sense of personal threat lead to a need to escape or run, generating the setting for constant hyperventilation and autonomic excitability. Such a sense of personal vulnerability or imminent danger may be similar to the sense of physical inadequacy among the group of "hysterical" subjects described by Lowry (1967).

The syndrome may simply be a learned behavior in some otherwise healthy individuals or learned only among subjects with the preceding forms of vulnerability. Lum notes that the thoracic breathing pattern is a diagnostic hallmark of the syndrome. The thoracic or sternal breathing pattern may be "learned" in fulfillment of certain role models. In men it may be a symbol of virility and a warning against aggression. In women, thoracic breathing draws attention to the bosom as a sexual symbol (Lum, 1975). Among obsessional people with phobic traits, such learned behavior is particularly likely. As a history of respiratory illness may be present in as many as 50% of subjects with episodic hyperventilation, the tendency to anticipate ventilatory insufficiency at times of stress may represent a learned behavior which continues long after the respiratory illness is corrected (Rice, 1950; Pfeffer, 1978; Lum, 1975).

EXAGGERATED VENTILATORY DRIVE

Ames noted that, although stress was a cause of overbreathing in most subjects as "a preparation for motor activity," hyperventilation resulted from a stimulus to an automatic respiratory center which remained in some way autonomous from conscious control. The central neuronal regulation of breathing and response to arterial gases involves several primarily brain stem and hypothalamic mechanisms, but a participating role of cortex or subcortical structures remains undemonstrated (Berger et al., 1977). The initial ventilatory response to either vigorous exercise or stress actually precedes skeletal muscle activation (Jensen et al., 1971), probably too rapidly to be due to conscious mechanisms. Peripheral and central chemoreceptors should be expected to cause inhibition of automatic respiratory centers (Farber and Bedell, 1973; Bicher et al., 1973; Berger et al., 1977) unless there were a superceding, probably automatic, stress-dependent stimulus.

Central neural feedback mechanisms respond quite differently to hypocapnia or alkalosis which results from active hyperventilation than they do to passive hyperventilation capable of causing marked hypocapnia and alkalosis; when passive overbreathing was stopped, animals remained apneic for variable periods until pH balance was restored. By contrast, in anesthetized animals induced to hyperventilate by either strong cutaneous stimuli or direct brain stem stimulation, there was no apneic interval when the stimulus was removed (Eldridge, 1977). In fact, the tidal volume and ventilatory rate did not return immediately to baseline normal levels but declined only gradually from the increased rate or volume—even in the face of continued hypocapnia and alkalosis. Eldridge also demonstrated that brain stem afterdischarges from the phrenic nerve continued to an exaggerated degree after removal of a stimulus inducing hyperventilation. Others have shown that when awake humans seldom have a posthyperventilation apnea and only gradually drop the tidal volume and breathing rate to baseline levels. In other words, once initiated, active hyperventilation seems to have a central basis of feedback reinforcement (Plum et al., 1962; Eldridge, 1977).

DIAGNOSIS OF HYPERVENTILATION

One important way in which the hyperventilation attack can be distinguished from the epileptic seizure is the tendency for hyperventilation attacks to cause different types of symptoms referable to different organ systems on different occasions (Pincus, 1978; Lum, 1975; McKell and Sullivan, 1947; Lewis, 1954). Perhaps the most telling diagnostic clue, however, is the *pattern of respiration*. Breathing may not occur at a more rapid than normal rate, but there is a particular breathing pattern. There is a heaving of upper sternum, which is often puzzling to the examiner in that it appears virtually effortless, and a lack of lateral costal expansion as might occur with normal chest breathing. This movement is the same as that employed in the normal sigh and Lum has emphasized that frequent sighing often precedes a hyperventilation attack. This pattern may become habitual, with most subjects being unconscious of their frequent sighing. The complete remission of symptoms by having the patient rebreathe his or her exhaled breath may also be diagnostic; however, it must be remembered that subjects whose epileptic seizures are triggered by hypocapnia may also have spells aborted by rebreathing and correcting the hypocapnia.

CNS lesions may cause rapid and deep respirations and may lead to profound respiratory alkalosis. Brain stem lesions affecting dorsal mid-brain tegmentum or pons may be particularly prone to cause hyperventilation. Increased intracranial pressure, perhaps by inducing midbrain compression, may also cause overbreathing. In such cases, lateral rib cage expansion and abdominal breathing movements, rather than the "sighing" quality characteristic of recurrent hyperventilation, are prominent features of the breathing efforts. The physiologic manifestations and symptoms of hyperventilation secondary to brain disease are the same as those due to anxiety-induced hyperventilation attacks. For this reason, due consideration of associated neurological disease and detailed neurological examination must be included in the evaluation of the subject with symptomatic hyperventilation. Other conditions such as drug ingestion (salicylates) or liver disease may also induce recurrent hyperventilation.

Hyperventilation is widely recognized as a precipitant of some forms of seizures; complex partial seizures or seizures arising from insular cortex may occasionally cause overbreathing as an ictal manifestation. In such cases, there are usually associated motor automatisms and blunting of consciousness and the breathing is more forced and usually involves abdominal muscles.

Most anxiety attacks or symptoms of cardiac or pulmonary insufficiency can be triggered by activity or anxiety. By contrast, attacks of hyperventilation, even those clearly due to psychogenic triggers, tend to occur when the patient is at rest (Lewis, 1953). Since most physicians anticipate that hyperventilation attacks might be triggered either by vigorous exercise or by anxiety, a spell that occurs when the patient is apparently at rest and not under stress is often not suspected of being due to a condition which could be of "psychogenic origin." The rapid deep breathing that occurs with exercise is compensatory and hence does not lead to hypocapnia and symptoms seen with spontaneous hyperventilation.

All authorities have emphasized that diagnostic confirmation of hyperventilation as a cause of symptoms may be obtained by reproducing one of the patient's spells with voluntary overbreathing. However, the symptoms of the attack depend not only on hypocapnia but also on an attendant degree of apprehension or anxiety which may be difficult to produce intentionally in the physician's office.

THE CHRONIC HYPERVENTILATION SYNDROME

Lewis (1953, 1954) argued that although acute hyperventilation attacks are easily detected, chronic hyperventilation syndromes are probably more common. They "masquerade behind symptoms referable to localized systems and are less often recognized." Many people are prone to chronic overbreathing. Many depressed patients have chronically increased tidal volumes and low arterial pCO_2 hovering on the brink of hypocapnia; they are subject to symptoms with even a slight increase in tidal volume or respiration rate. When stressed, only slight changes in their already exaggerated breathing patterns are needed to drop arterial pCO_2 sufficiently to produce symptoms. In a series of 50 patients with chronic hyperventilation, Lewis (1953, 1954) found CNS symptoms in 9 patients, and peripheral motor or sensory symptoms which others might have interpreted as CNS in origin in another 8 patients. Such symptoms were much more commonly seen in the "chronic syndrome" than in the acute form of hyperventilation syndrome.

Treatment of the acute hyperventilation attack consists of reassurance and rebreathing exhaled air, most conveniently performed with a small paper bag. When an underlying stress or neurosis can be identified, treatment may result in improvement of the overbreathing spells. Treatment of depression, often with tricyclic compounds, may significantly improve symptoms in some patients. For the patients with chronic hyperventilation syndrome, however, for whom overbreathing may be a learned behavior, treatment is limited. Often the patient must carry a paper bag to have available for rebreathing to "break the cycle" of accelerating hyperventilation in acute attacks.

Syncope and hyperventilation are probably the most common episodic disorders of consciousness to be confused with epileptic seizures. While in classic form the two phenomena ought to be easily distinguished from seizures, the autonomic manifestations of some seizures on one hand and the motor and sensory features of hyperventilation on the other hand make the distinction very difficult in many cases. Diagnosis depends upon awareness of subtle features of the two conditions and very often can be made only by witnessing or provoking a characteristic attack.

References

SYNCOPE

Abboud, F.M., Heistad, D.D., Mark, A.L., and Schmid, P.G. Reflex control of the peripheral circulation. *Progr. Cardiovasc. Dis.* 18:371–403, 1976.

Alicandri, C., Fouad, F.M., Tarazi, R.C., Castle, L., and Morant, V. Three cases of hypotension and syncope with ventricular pacing: Possible role of atrial reflexes. *Am. J. Cardiol.* 42:137–142, 1978.

Aviado, D.M., and Schmidt, C.F. Cardiovascular and respiratory reflexes from the left side of the heart. *Am. J. Physiol.* 196:726, 1959.

Barlow, J.B., and Pocock, W.A. Mitral valve prolapse: The specific billowing mitral leaflet syndrome or an insignificant nonejection systolic click. *Am Heart J.* 97:277–283, 1979.

Bergenwald, L., Freyschuss, U., and Sjostrand, T. The mechanism of orthostatic and hemorrhagic fainting. *Scand. J. Clin. Lab. Invest.* 37:209–217, 1977.

Bichat, X. *Recherches Physiologique sur la vie et la Mort,* ed. 3. Brosson, Gabon, et Cie, Paris, 1805.

Blumenthal, M.D., and Davie, J.W. Dizziness and falling in elderly physiatric out-patients. *Am. J. Psychiatry* 137:203–206, 1980.

Boudoulas, H., Dalmangas, G., Schaal, S.F., and Lewis, R.P. Superiority of 24-hour monitoring for evaluation of syncope. *Circulation 54 (suppl 2):9,* 1976.

Boudoulas, H., Schaal, S.F., Lewis, R.P., and Robinson, J.L. Superiority of 24-hour out-patient monitoring over multi-stage exercise testing for the evaluation of syncope. *J. Electrocardiol.* 12(1):103–108, 1979.

Braunwald, E. *Heart Disease: A Textbook of Cardiovascular Medicine.* Saunders, Philadelphia, 1980, pp. 956–961.

Brick, J.E. Cold water syncope. *South. Med. J.* 71:1579–1580, 1978.

Caffi, J. Zur Frage klinischer Anfallformen bei psychomotorischer Epilepsie. *Schweiz. Med. Wochenschr.* 103:469–475, 1973.

Clark, P.I., Glasser, S.P., and Spoto, E. Arrhythmias detected by ambulatory monitoring. *Chest* 77:722–725, 1979.

Davies, A.B., Stephens, M.R., and Davies, A.G. Carotid sinus hypersensitivity in patients presenting with syncope. *Br. Heart J.* 42:583–586, 1979.

Delgado-Escueta, A.V. Epileptogenic paroxysms: Modern approaches and clinical correlations. *Neurology* 29:1014–1022, 1979.

Devereux, R.B., Perloff, J.K., Reicihek, N., and Josephson, M.E. Mitral valve prolapse. *Circulation* 54:3–8, 1976.

Dodge, P.R., Richardson, E.P., and Victor, M. Recurrent convulsive seizures as a sequel to cerebral infarction. *Brain* 77:610–638, 1954.

Donker, D.E., Medina, R., and Kieft, J. Micturition syncope. *Electroencephalogr. Clin. Neurophysiol.* 33:328–331, 1972.

Duvoisin, R.C. Convulsive syncope induced by the Weber maneuver. *Arch. Neurol.* 7:219–221, 1962.

Eckberg, D.L., Drabinsky, M., and Braunwald, E. Defective cardiac parasympathetic control in patients with heart disease. *N. Engl. J. Med.* 285:877–883, 1971.

Edmonson, H.D. Vasovagal episodes in the dental surgery. *J. Dent.* 6(3):189–195, 1978.

Engel, G.L., and Romano, J. Studies of syncope: IV. Biologic interpretation of vasodepressor syncope. *Psychosom. Med.* 9:288–294, 1947.

Engel, G.L., Romano, J., and McLin, T. Vasodepressor and carotid sinus syncope: EEG, ECG, and clinical observations. *Arch. Intern. Med.* 74:100–119, 1944.

Engel, G.L. *Fainting.* Charles C Thomas, Springfield, IL, 1962.

Engel, G.L. Psychologic stress, vasodepressor (vasovagal) syncope and sudden death. *Ann. Intern. Med.* 89:403–412, 1978.

Ewing, D.J., Campbell, I.W., and Clarke, B.F. Assessment of cardiovascular effects in diabetic autonomic neuropathy and prognostic implications. *Ann. Intern. Med.* 92(suppl):308–311, 1980.

Ferris, E.B., Capps, R.B., and Weiss, S. Carotid sinus syncope. *Medicine* 14:377–456, 1934.

Gastaut, H. Syncope, generalized anoxic seizures. In *Handbook of Clinical Neurology,* edited by Vinken, P.J., and Bruyn, G.W. *The Epilepsies,* vol. 15. Elsevier, Amsterdam, 1974.

Gastaut, H., and Fischer-Williams, M. Electroencephalographic study of syncope: Its differentiation from epilepsy. *Lancet* 7004:1018–1025, 1957.

Gastaut, H., and Gastaut, Y. Electroencephalographic study of anoxic convulsions in childhood. *Electroencephalogr. Clin. Neurophysiol.* 10:607–620, 1958.

Gastaut, H., and Meyer, J.S. *Cerebral Anoxia and the Electroencephalogram.* Charles C Thomas, Springfield, IL, 1961.

Gowers, W.R. *Epilepsy and Chronic Convulsive Diseases: Their Causes, Symptoms, and Treatment,* ed. 2. London, Churchill, 1901.

Graham, D.T., Kabler, J.D., and Lunsford, L. Vasovagal fainting: A diphasic response. *Psychosom. Med.* 23:493–507, 1961.

Jacobson, R.R. Glosso-pharyngeal neuralgia with cardiac arrhythmia: A rare but treatable cause of syncope. *Br. Med. J. 1(6160)*:379–380, 1979.

Lesser, L.M., and Wenger, N.K. Carotid sinus syncope. *Heart Lung 5*:453–456, 1976.

Lloyd-Smith, W. and Tatlow, J. *Electroencephalogr. Clin. Neurophysiol. 10*:153, 1953.

Luxon, L.M., Crowther, A., Harrison, M.J., and Coltart, D.J. Controlled study of 24-hour ambulatory ECG monitoring in patients with transient neurologic symptoms. *J. Neurol. Neurosurg. Psychiatry 43*:37–41, 1980.

Mills, P., Ross, J., Hollingsworth, J., Amara, I., and Craig, E. Long term prognosis of mitral valve prolapse. *N. Engl. J. Med. 297*:13–17, 1979.

Mutani, M. EEG features in syncope. *Minerva Med. 62*:2518, 1971.

Plum, F. Cardiac arrhythmias and neurological dysfunction, pp. 11–20. In *Cerebral Manifestations of Episodic Cardiac Dysrhythmias*, edited by Busse, E.W. Excerpta Medica, Amsterdam, 1979.

Pocock, W.A., and Barlow, J.B. Post-exercise arrhythmias in the billowing mitral leaflet syndrome. *Am. Heart J. 80*:740–746, 1976.

Pomerantz, B., and O'Rourke, R.A. The Stokes-Adams syndrome. *Am. J. Med. 46*:941–960, 1969.

Rees, J.R. Glossopharyngeal neuralgia with syncope. *Br. Med. J 1(6165)*:754, 1979.

Riley, T.L. Ischemic neurapraxia of the vocal cords. *South. Med. J. 74*:229–230, 1981.

Riley, T.L., and Berndt, T., The role of the EEG technologist in delineating pseudoseizures. *Am. J. EEG Technol. 20*:89–96, 1980.

Riley, T.L., and Friedman, J.M. Strokes, orthostatic hypotension, and focal seizures. *J.A.M.A. 245*:1243–1244, 1981.

Romano, J., and Engel, G.L. Studies of syncope: III. Differentiation between vasodepressor and hysterical fainting. *Psychosom. Med. 7*:3–15, 1945.

Schott, G.D., McLead, A.A., and Jewitt, D.E. Cardiac arrhythmias that masquerade as epilepsy. *Br. Med. J. 1*:1454–1457, 1979.

Sledge, W.H., and Boydstun, J.A. Vasovagal syncope in aircrews. *J. Nerv. Ment. Dis. 167*: 114–124, 1979.

Stephenson, J.B.P. Non-epileptic television syncope. *Br. Med. J. 1*:1622, 1978.

Sutton, R., and Perrins, E.J. Neurologic manifestations of the sick sinus syndrome, pp. 174–184. In *Cerebral Manifestations of Episodic Cardiac Dysrhythmia*. edited by Busse, E.W. Excerpta Medica, Amsterdam, 1977.

Tabatsnik, B. Holter recording stakes out three clinical areas. *Clin. Trends Cardiol. 6*:6–7, 1976.

Taylor, P.H. Glossopharyngeal neuralgia with syncope. *J. Laryngol. Otol. 91*:859–868, 1977.

Walter, P.F., Reid, S.D., and Wenger, N.K. Transient cerebral ischemia due to arrhythmia. *Ann. Intern. Med. 72*:471–474, 1970.

Watkins, P.J., and MacKay, J.D. Cardiac denervation in diabetic neuropathy. *Ann. Intern. Med. 92 (suppl)*:304–307, 1980.

Winkle, R.A., Lopes, M.G., Fitzgerald, J.W., Goodman, D.J., Schroeder, J.S., and Harrison, D.C. Arrhythmias in patients with mitral valve prolapse. *Circulation 52*:73–77, 1975.

Ziegler, D.K., Lin, J., and Bayer, W.L. Convulsive syncope: Relationship to cerebral ischemia. *Trans. Am. Neurol. Assoc. 103*:150–154, 1978.

HYPERVENTILATION

Adams, J.E., and Severinghaus, J.W. Oxygen tension of human cerebral grey and white matter: The effects of hyperventilation. *J. Neurosurg. 19*:959–963, 1962.

Ames, F. The hyperventilation syndrome. *J. Ment. Sci. 101*:468–525, 1955.

Berger, A.J., Mitchel, R.A., and Severinghaus, J.W. Regulations of respiration *N. Engl. J. Med. 297*:92–97, 138–143, 194–201 (three parts), 1977.

Bicher, H.I., Reneau, D.D., Bruly, D.F., and Kinsley, H. Brain oxygen supply and neuronal activity under normal and hypoglycemic conditions. *Am. J. Physiol. 224*:275–285, 1973

Burns, B.H., and Howell, J.B. Disproportionately severe breathlessness in chronic bronchitis *Q. Med. J. 38*:277–294, 1969.

Damas Mora, J.D. The effect of mild hyperventilation on red cell sodium. *Br. J. Psychiatry* 130:459–462, 1977.

Damas Mora, J.D., Grant, L., Kenyon, P., and Patel, M.K. Respiratory ventilation and carbon dioxide levels in syndromes of depression. *Br. J. Psychiatry* 129:457–464, 1976.

Davis, H., and Wallace, W.M. Factors affecting changes produced in electrencephalogram by standardized hyperventilation. *Arch. Neurol. Psychol.* 57:606–625, 1942.

DuLaurens, A. *A Discourse of the Preservation of the Sight; of Melancholie Diseases; of Rheumes; and of Old Age.* London, 1559.

Eldridge, F.L. Central neural respiratory stimulatory effect of active respiration. *J. Appl. Physiol.* 37:723–735, 1974.

Eldridge, F.L. Maintenance of respiration by central neural feedback mechanisms. *Fed. Proc.* 36:2400–2404, 1977.

Engel, G. A reconsideration of the role of conversion of somatic disease. *Compr. Psychiatry* 9:316–326, 1968.

Engel, G.L., Ferriss, E.B., and Logan, M. Hyperventilation: Analysis of clinical symptomology. *Ann. Intern. Med.* 27:683–704, 1947.

Farber, J.P., and Bedell, G.N. Responsiveness of breathing control centers to CO_2 and neurogenic stimuli. *Respir. Physiol.* 19:88–95, 1973.

Fraser, R., and Sargent, W. Hyperventilation attacks: Manifestation in hysteria. *Br. Med. J.* 1:378–380, 1938.

Gibbs, E.L., Lennox, W.G., and Gibbs, F.A. Variations of carbon dioxide content of blood in epilepsy. *Arch. Neurol. Psychol.* 43:223–241, 1940.

Gliebe, P.A., and Auerbach, A. Sighing and other forms of hyperventilation simulating organic disease. *J. Nerv. Ment. Dis.* 99:600–615, 1944.

Goldman, A. Clinical tetany by forced respiration. *J.A.M.A.* 78:1193, 1922.

Gotoh, F., Meyer, J.S., and Takagi, Y. Cerebral effects of hyperventilation in man. *Arch Neurol* 12:410–423, 1965.

Gottlieb, B. Nonorganic disease in medical out-patients. *Med. Update* 1:917–922, 1969.

Grant, S.B., Goldman, A. A study of forced respiration: Experimental production of tetany. *Am. J. Physiol.* 52:209–232, 1920–1921.

Haldane, J.S., and Poulton, E.P. The effects of want of oxygen on respiration. *J. Physiol.* 37:390–410, 1908.

Henderson, Y. Acapnia and shock: VI. Fatal apnea after excessive respiration. *Am. J. Physiol.* 25:310–333, 1909–1910.

Hill, L., and Flack, M. The influence of oxygen inhalators on muscular work. *J. Physiol.* 40:347–372, 1910.

Jensen, J.I., Vejby-Christensen, H., and Petersen, E.S. Ventilation in man at onset of work employing different standardized starting orders. *Respir. Physiol.* 13:209–220, 1971.

Joorabachi, B. Expressions of hyperventilation syndrome in children. *Clin. Pediatr.* 16:1110–1115, 1977.

Kennealy, J.A., McLennan, J.E., Loudon, R.G., and McLaurin, R.L. Hyperventilation-induced cerebral hypoxia *Am. Rev. Respir. Dis.* 122:407–417, 1980.

Kerr, W.J., Dalton, W., and Gliebe, P.A. Some physical phenomena associated with anxiety states and their relation to hyperventilation. *Ann. Intern. Med.* 2:961–992, 1937.

Kety, S.S., Schmidt, C.F. The effects of active and passive hyperventilation on cerebral blood flow, cerebral oxygen consumption, cardiac output and blood pressure of normal young men. *J. Clin. Invest.* 25:107–119, 1946.

Lassen, N.A. Brain extracellular fluid pH: The main factor controlling cerebral blood flow. *Scand. J. Lab. Clin.* 2:247–251, 1968.

Lazarus, H.R., and Kostan, J.J. Psychogenic hyperventilation and death anxiety. *Psychosomatics* 10:14–22, 1969.

Lewis, B.I. The hyperventilation syndrome. *Ann. Intern. Med.* 38:918–927, 1953.

Lewis, B.I. Chronic hyperventilation syndrome. *J.A.M.A.* 155:1204–1208, 1954.

Lowry, T.P. *Hyperventilation and Hysteria.* Charles C Thomas, Springfield, IL, 1967.

Lum, L.C. Hyperventilation: The tip and the iceberg, *J. Psychosom. Res.* 19:325–383, 1975.

McKell, T.E., and Sullivan, A.D. The hyperventilation syndrome in gastroenterology.

Gastroenterology 9:6–16, 1947.

Pfeffer, J.M. The aetiology of the hyperventilation syndrome. *Psychother. Psychosom. 30*: 47–55, 1978.

Pincus, J.H. Disorders of conscious awareness: Hyperventilation syndrome. *Br. J. Hosp. Med. 19*:312–313, 1978.

Plum, F., Brown, H.W., and Snoep, E. Neurologic significance of posthyperventilation apnea. *J.A.M.A. 181*:1050–1055, 1962.

Plum, F., and Posner, J.B. *Diagnosis of Stupor and Coma.* F.A. Davis, Philadelphia, 1972.

Raichle, M.E., Posner, J.B., and Plum, F. Cerebral blood flow during and after hyperventilation. *Arch. Neurol. 23*:394–403, 1970.

Raichle, M.E., and Plum, F. Hyperventilation and cerebral blood flow. *Stroke 3*:566–575, 1972.

Reivich, M. Arterial PCO_2 and cerebral hemodynamics. *Am. J. Physiol. 206*:25–35, 1964.

Rice, R. Symptom patterns of the hyperventilation syndrome. *Am. J. Med. 8*:691–700, 1950.

Rosett, J. The experimental production of rigidity, nonvoluntary movements and of abnormal states of consciousness. *Brain 47*:294–336, 1942.

Stead, E.A., and Warren, J.V. Clinical significance of hyperventilation. *Am. J. Med. Sci. 206*:183–190, 1943.

White, P.D., and Hahn, R.G. Symptom of sighing in cardiovascular diagnosis: With observations *Am. J. Med. Sci. 177*:179–188, 1929.

Chapter 4 Narcolepsy

J. DAVID PARKES, F.R.C.P., D.P.M.

A Japanese legend tells of a priest who came from India to China in AD 519 and who succumbed to sleep when he wished to watch and pray. In a moment of anger he cut off his two eyelids which changed into a shrub, a tea tree, whose leaves are eminently calculated to prevent sleep. Unfortunately for those people who readily believe legends in whole or in part, the Chinese have never heard of this story.* Whatever the truth of the matter, irresistible sleep has altered the course of history and mention must be made of the soldiers who slept during the resurrection of Christ, King Alfred who burnt the cakes and Napoleon who slept for 36 hours after his defeat at the battle of Aspern. In China the herb Ma Huang (Ephedra Vulgaris) was used as a stimulant 5000 years ago, although more recently considered as too toxic for clinical use. In attempting to make a synthetic substitute for ephedrine, Gordon Alles synthesized amphetamine in 1927.

NARCOLEPSY, CATAPLEXY AND EPILEPSY

Narcolepsy and cataplexy are not usually confused with epilepsy, although they have been considered as seizure disorders. In both narcolepsy and epilepsy there is a change in awareness, although in narcolepsy this is physiologic in nature and unlike the situation in epilepsy. A number of brain diseases will cause both conditions, although often these are not associated with any known structural or biochemical disorder. In narcolepsy, fits do not occur and seizure activity is absent from the EEG. Cataplexy may be confused with drop attacks or atonic episodes but the first condition is usually triggered by a sudden change in arousal with laughter, emotion, surprise or stress, whilst banal drop attacks in middle-aged women or atonic episodes with petit mal usually have no definitive precipitant. Antiepileptic drugs are not of value in narcolepsy.

---

* De Candolle. *Origin of Cultivated Plants.* Kegan Paul Trench, London, 1886.

Diagnostic difficulties occur mostly in children who suddenly fall or drop asleep whilst at school. The correct diagnosis can almost always be made if an attack is witnessed. Gowers (1907) considered narcolepsy in the borderland of epilepsy, although he clearly distinguished between the two conditions and stressed that, whereas in epilepsy most attacks are unpredictable, narcolepsy usually results from monotony and cataplexy from surprise. Narcolepsy and cataplexy can thus be viewed as normal physiological events with predictable occurrence in subjects with a disturbance in arousal in contrast to the nonphysiological nature of epilepsy. The abnormality in narcolepsy lies in the frequency rather than in the nature of attack.

DEVELOPMENT OF CONCEPTS OF NARCOLEPSY AND CATAPLEXY

Narcolepsy was first clearly defined in Europe in the last decades of the 19th century (Table 4.1), although Thomas Willis, Professor of Physics, had recognized the condition in restoration Oxford as early as 1660 and Oliver in 1704 described the case of an extraordinary sleepy person at Timsberg, near Bath. Sleeping sickness, a disease considered confined to black people, had been seen in Africa by early slave traders

Table 4.1
Development of Concepts of Narcolepsy*

Descriptive neurology	1850–1900. Gélineau, Westphal, de Manaceine and many others describe sleep disorders
Encephalitis lethargica	1917–1927. Symonds and Adie describe narcolepsy following encephalitis lethargica
Narcoleptic syndrome	1920–1940. Wilson, Daniels, Lhermitte and others describe classic features of narcoleptic tetrad
Diagnostic criteria	1957. Yoss and Daly establish clinical criteria for diagnosis
EEG criteria	1957. Aserinsky and Kleitman discover REM sleep 1960. Premature onset of REM sleep in narcoleptics described by Vogel
Sleep laboratory studies	1960–1980. Dramatic increase in knowledge of sleep disorders and study of sleep apnea, narcolepsy variants and hypersomnolence

* After Passouant, 1976.

and sea captains, and sleep disorders were at one time thought to only occur in blacks (Passouant, 1976). However, many apparently different states of altered awareness, including trance, hypersomnolence, automatic behavior, sleep walking, hypnosis and narcolepsy, were described in white subjects at the end of the 19th century. In addition to these sleep disorders, changes in muscle tone with epidemics of muscle rigidity were also described, such as that occurring in Billinghausen, near Würzburg, and which affected half the inhabitants who became pale with motionless limbs and fixed postures (De Manaceine, 1897).

The French neuropsychiatrist Gelineau brought order to these accounts and introduced the term "narcolepsy" (derived from the Greek *narke*, meaning somnolence, and *lepsis*, a seizure) to describe the condition of a dealer in hogsheads who had many attacks of intense sleep each day as well as episodic loss of muscle tone, usually caused by laughter (Gelineau, 1880). This condition was named "cataplexy" by Henneberg (1916) in distinction from catalepsy which was accompanied by increase in muscle tone and resulted in a fixed posture that could be maintained for long periods without fatigue. Both disorders were accompanied by paralysis of movement, although only catalepsy was frequently associated with epilepsy or hysteria.

Cataplexy was recognized as being closely similar to sleep paralysis, a borderline normal event. Both conditions and also narcolepsy were considered as excessively rare and Gowers claimed that for every 15 cases of narcolepsy 30,000 cases of epilepsy would come under observation (1907).

The worldwide epidemic of encephalitis lethargica between 1917 and 1927 was followed by a severe sleep disturbance in many cases (Symonds, 1926). However, it was apparent that most people with narcolepsy did not have a history of encephalitis or other brain disease. There was considerable controversy as to whether narcolepsy was a disease in its own right or was merely a symptom of many different conditions and possibly resulting from pituitary or other deficiency (Adie, 1926).

Between 1920 and 1950 the frequency, genetic basis and exact clinical features of narcolepsy and the narcoleptic syndrome were carefully defined, largely from studies at The Mayo Clinic (Yoss and Daly, 1957). The next landmark was the recognition of REM sleep and the discovery that the timing of this was abnormal in some patients with sleep disturbance (Aserinsky and Kleitman, 1953; Vogel, 1960; Rechtschaffen et al., 1963; Takahashi and Jimbo, 1963). The subsequent development of sleep laboratories in America and Europe has led to a great increase in understanding the disorders of excessive sleep, although the biochemical basis for narcolepsy still has not been determined.

CLINICAL DEFINITIONS

Narcolepsy

Narcolepsy is excessive daytime sleepiness, often occurring under unusual circumstances such as whilst standing, eating, talking, traveling and even during sexual relations.

Hypersomnolence

Recurrent daytime sleepiness is referred to as hypersomnolence. Although sleep attacks may occur, these are not as sudden, as irresistible or as refreshing as in narcolepsy. Patients often feel constantly tired. The condition may be isolated or familial and is not accompanied by early onset of REM activity during night sleep.

Narcoleptic Syndrome (Synonyms: Narcolepsy and Cataplexy, Narcoleptic Tetrad)

The combination of narcolepsy with cataplexy is characteristic and unique. Sleep paralysis, automatic behavior and hypnagogic hallucinations are important accessory symptoms, although not occurring in all patients. The frequency with which these symptoms are associated may be largely dependent on the thoroughness of history or accuracy of witnessed accounts. The approximate frequency is as follows:

1. Narcolepsy, cataplexy and one other associated symptom: 20–30%
2. Narcolepsy, cataplexy, sleep paralysis, hypnagogic hallucinations: 30–40%.†

The narcoleptic syndrome is characterized by the appearance of REM sleep within 10 minutes of sleep onset.

Cataplexy

Cataplexy is the loss of muscle tone with paralysis of voluntary movement accompanied by areflexia, almost always triggered by surprise, emotion and, in particular, laughter. The severity and duration of attacks may vary widely. Awareness is usually maintained.

Sleep Paralysis

Voluntary muscle paralysis, sometimes accompanied by respiratory embarrassment, occurring at the start or end of sleep is referred to as sleep paralysis. The patient may lose all sense of the passage of time but most attacks last only a few minutes. Sleep paralysis is often

---

† Data from King's College Hospital and Maudsley patients. Other series show a variable degree of symptom association.

accompanied by vivid dreams and sometimes illusions of weightlessness or flying. Unlike cataplexy, sleep paralysis is not triggered by external stimuli.

Automatic Behavior

Automatic behavior is lapse of memory, blackouts, trance or sleep-walking in which new complex behavior may be faulty but simple reflex behavior is usually normal. There is subsequent amnesia for the period of automatic behavior.

Hypnagogic Hallucinations

Vivid perceptual dreamlike experiences at sleep onset or on waking (hypnopompic) are referred to as hypnagogic hallucinations.

Obstructive Sleep Apnea

Obstructive sleep apnea is manifest by multiple periods (up to 200) of apnea during sleep, often with gross snoring, sleep restlessness and excessive daytime drowsiness.

Sleep Drunkenness

Impairment of normal awareness for prolonged periods after waking, sometimes with automatic behavior, is referred to as sleep drunkenness.

Normal Sleep Habits

Sleep with monotony and weakness with laughter are normal events. A small percentage of normal subjects have an infrequent attack of sleep paralysis, and dreams at sleep onset are not an uncommon experience. Infrequent respiratory pauses occur during normal sleep.

Because of these normal symptoms, the diagnosis and classification of excessive day sleep and associated symptoms remain unsatisfactory despite the publication of useful guidelines (Association of Sleep Disorders Centers, 1979). In the majority of conditions described, examination is completely normal and, therefore, diagnosis is dependent on an accurate history, if necessary assisted by polygraphic studies.

PATHOLOGY

Primary Narcolepsy

Many different diseases of the brain cause a disturbance of awareness. The anatomical localization rather than the etiology of the lesion is important in determining the effect on sleep. In most people with narcolepsy, there are no signs of organic brain disease although there may be a functional disorder of brain stem reticular formation activity. Narcolepsy and continuous cataplexy have been described in patients with tumors of the major reticular formation nucleus, the locus ceruleus (Jouvet and Delorme, 1965). A high concentration of noradrenaline occurs in this area of the brain but there is no evidence of a generalized defect of noradrenaline synthesis or release in narcoleptics.

The nature of sleep disturbance is usually different in primary and secondary narcolepsy, which may be characterized by reversal of sleep rhythms or persistent hypersomnolence rather than periodic day sleep as well as by signs of focal brain disease (Table 4.2).

Secondary Narcolepsy

Mauthner in 1890 described anatomically localized lesions in the periventricular gray matter and in neighboring parts of the diencephalon and mesencephalon in patients with sleep disorders. He showed that many focal or diffuse structural lesions that impinge on the mechanisms of consciousness will result in pathological changes in awareness. Mauthner assumed that drowsiness was due to involvement of the mesencephalon and diencephalon, and it became customary to describe these as Mauthner's area.

Table 4.2
Primary and Secondary Sleep Disorders*, †

Primary	
Narcoleptic syndrome	Early onset REM
Narcolepsy alone	Early onset REM
Hypersomnolence	Non-REM
Secondary	
Sleep apnea	Central or peripheral cause with polygraphic changes
Encephalitis lethargica	Encephalitic illness with subsequent sleep reversal, narcolepsy or hypersomnolence
Brain stem encephalitis	
Generalized encephalitis	
Head injury	Focal brain injury
Salivary tumor around carotid sheath	Disturbance of cerebral blood flow
Disseminated sclerosis	Uncertain association
Midline brain tumors	Involvement reticular nucleii or projection
Trypanosomiasis	Paraventricular pathology with disturbed sleep rhythms in terminal illness
Pickwickian syndrome	Obesity, apnea, CO_2 retention
Klein-Levin syndrome	Prolonged periodic hypersomnolence with hyperphagia

* Sleep disturbance is dependent on the site and not the nature of the pathology.

† After Parkes and Marsden, 1974.

Encephalitis

Following the worldwide epidemic of encephalitis lethargica in 1917–1927, many patients developed a condition resembling narcolepsy and Daniel's analysis of the Mayo Clinic records (1934) showed that most patients with postencephalitic narcolepsy also had a condition resembling cataplexy. As examples, Symonds (1926) described a native of Iceland with postencephalitic parkinsonism who fell whenever he laughed, with a little twitching of the facial muscles; Bonhoeffer (1928) described a similar patient without definite narcolepsy but with periodic weakness of the facial and neck muscles. Periodic somnolence rather than narcolepsy accompanied by hypnagogic hallucinations but not cataplexy following an encephalitic illness was described by Pohl (1966). Postmortem findings in this 52-year-old man showed ill-defined inflammatory changes in the posterior paramedian regions of the periventricular gray matter of the thalamus. Previously, the work of Von Economo and Grippe (1919) had stressed the importance of lesions in the caudal part of the third ventricle and brain stem.

Other Causes of Excessive Sleep

Many different structural lesions other than encephalitis have been associated with sleep disorder. These include neoplasms, particularly those around the aqueduct and ventricles, tumors of the pineal and hypothalamus, brain stem and third ventricle, as well as those causing raised intracerebral pressure; many different vascular diseases, including vertebrobasilar insufficiency and multi-infarct dementia; infective conditions such as brain abscess and syphilis; and a number of degenerative disorders, including senile dementia and Alzheimer's disease. Single patients with narcolepsy associated with disseminated sclerosis, cerebellar tumor, temporal lobe epilepsy, familial tremor, peptic ulcer and congenital ocular pareses have been described (Association of Sleep Disorders Centers, 1979; Parkes and Marsden, 1974); these associations may largely be due to chance. In addition to this wealth of structural lesions, many functional disorders, personality disorders, hypochondriasis, schizophrenia, the use and abuse of drugs, alcohol or drug withdrawal, different endocrine disorders, uremia, hypercapnia, liver failure, miscellaneous pyrexial states and anemia will all result in excessive daytime sleep.

PHYSIOLOGY

Narcolepsy

Lombard (1887—in de Manaceine, 1897) examined normal people during sleep and described loss of muscle tone and reflexes during certain sleep phases. He made the repeated observation that a dream of active movement was associated with a very violent knee kick. During the same period, Rosenbach (1881—in de Manceine, 1897) systematically observed the reflexes excited in children by tickling the palm of the hand and the sole of the foot and the tendon reflexes during sleep and waking and found that flickering of the facial muscles, eye movements and occasional body movements occurred. Similar features accompany some but not all attacks of day sleep in narcoleptic subjects.

Cataplexy

As in some sleep phases, head movement, trembling, grimaces and tongue protrusion occasionally occur during both cataplexy and sleep paralysis. In addition cataplexy is sometimes accompanied by pallor, pupillary dilatation, sweating and increase in pulse rate, although these features may result from the surprise that usually initiates the attack. Wilson (1928) described atonia and areflexia with an extensor plantar response during an attack of cataplexy or sleep paralysis, and Mussio Fournio claimed that facial muscles were inexcitable by normal electrical stimulation during cataplexy (Parkes and Marsden, 1974).

Sleep Paralysis

Weir Mitchell in 1896 considered that sleep paralysis was a normal physiological event, the spell to be broken by an acute mental effort to move. Maury (1848) thought that, like sleep paralysis, hypnagogic hallucinations were a normal event. He described the whole range of visual imagery with luminous phenomena: flowers, landscapes, arabesques of geometrical figures that could be summoned but not controlled in the moments before falling asleep. To concentrate was to cause the vision to vanish. In contrast to these not unpleasant dreams, hallucinoses in narcoleptics sometimes have an especially vivid or horrific quality.

Rapid Eye Movement (REM) Sleep

REM sleep was discovered by Aserinsky and Kleitman in 1953. Vogel (1960) showed that the night sleep of narcoleptics began with an REM phase, a finding confirmed by Rechtschaffen et al. (1963) and by Takahashi and Jimbo (1963).

This discovery explained many features of the narcoleptic syndrome, for vivid dreams, atonia and paralysis of movement accompany REM sleep as well as narcolepsy and cataplexy.

EEG FINDINGS IN NARCOLEPSY

The premature onset of REM sleep which occurs at night does not always occur during daytime narcolepsy, although Hishikawa and his colleagues (1968) showed that narcoleptics fall asleep in the daytime with a shorter latency and spend more time asleep than do controls. In addition to early onset of REM periods, the night sleep of narcoleptics is often very disturbed, with many shifts of sleep phase and frequent awakenings.

Sleep onset REM periods are reported to occur between 49 and 100% of all patients with narcolepsy and cataplexy. The percentage of patients with at least one sleep onset REM period shown by one night's recording is approximately 50%; with two subsequent nights' recordings, 75%; and with three nights, 82%. If in addition daytime nap recordings are done, the percentage of patients with at least one sleep onset REM period is increased to about 95%.

In addition to the sleep onset REM periods, the sleep latency test is of value in the diagnosis of narcolepsy. Most subjects with the narcoleptic syndrome go to sleep within 2 to 3 minutes of lying down in a quieted room, as compared with a period of 10 to 20 minutes in normal subjects.

Whatever the EEG findings, a definite history of cataplexy accompanying narcolepsy indicates the clinical diagnosis of the narcoleptic syndrome.

Many patients with narcolepsy have nocturnal myoclonus with particular involvement of the lower limbs. This occasionally results in arousal and so may account, at least in part, for some increase in daytime drowsiness.

The timing and occurrence of REM sleep may be altered by laboratory habituation, posture, amphetamine treatment and drug withdrawal. These facts must be taken into consideration in the assessment of EEG recording in the diagnosis of narcolepsy.

The EEG shows no specific or diagnostic features during an attack of cataplexy or sleep paralysis. These are similar phenomena, distinguished only by the state immediately prior to their occurrence and the degree of awareness during the attack. During cataplexy, total awareness and a waking EEG are found in most patients although muscle tone, tendon reflexes and the H reflex are lost. These changes may be due to selective triggering of descending but not ascending REM systems, brought about by intense emotional stimuli and resulting in motor neurone inhibition but not eye movements or dreaming. During an attack of sleep paralysis this descending inhibitory system continues to function from the preceding REM phase, with dissociation of ascending and descending components of REM sleep. The patient is awake and a verbal stimulus can be recalled but a motor response may be difficult or impossible (Nan'no et al., 1970).

Hypnagogic hallucinations in narcoleptics are accompanied by REM activity and represent the dreams of this sleep phase. Cataplexy with subsequent dreaming and sleep paralysis immediately followed or accompanied by vivid dreams have both been recorded, and as with other features of the narcoleptic syndrome indicate the mistiming and dissociation of normal function in the ascending and descending REM systems.

CLINICAL FEATURES OF THE NARCOLEPTIC SYNDROME
(Table 4.3)

Frequency

The exact prevalence of narcolepsy in the United States and the United kingdom is not known, although many large case series have been described. However, recent estimates of 100,000 narcoleptics in the United States and perhaps 20,000 in the United Kingdom are based on comparatively small samples (Parkes and Marsden, 1974). An approximate estimate of the frequency is that there are 4 cases of narcolepsy per 10,000 of the population (Association of Sleep Disorders Centers, 1979). The condition is equally common in both sexes.

Genetics

Narcolepsy often occurs in families. Krabbe and Magnussen (1942) described a family in which 4 of 12 sibs had a sleep disorder and, reviewing other reports, found 54 narcoleptics belonging to 19 families. Using more exact diagnostic criteria, Yoss and Daly (1957) found that 30% of subjects with the narcoleptic syndrome had at least one affected relative. Narcolepsy or cataplexy alone may predominate in some fam-

Table 4.3
Clinical Features of the Narcoleptic Syndrome*

	Narcolepsy	Cataplexy	Sleep Paralysis	Hypnagogic Hallucinations
Age at onset (mean and range)	24 (5–66)	29 (9–66)	28 (9–50)	Uncertain
Frequency of attacks	5/day (1–20)	Very variable Less than one to over 100/week	Very variable but usually 8–10/year	Several times each night
Duration of attack	30 minutes (1–100, sometimes longer)	30 seconds (1 second– 60 minutes)	Around 2–3 minutes	Uncertain

* After Parkes et al, 1975.

ilies. Daly and Yoss (1959) described a family in which 12 members had narcolepsy over four generations; only 3 of the 12 had cataplexy. In contrast, Gelardi and Brown (1967) described a family in which 15 members had cataplexy, 3 had sleep paralysis, but only 3 had narcolepsy over three generations. Kessler et al. (1974) studied 50 subjects with narcolepsy and cataplexy, all with early onset REM sleep, of whom 52% had an affected relative either with narcolepsy alone or with the narcoleptic syndrome. There is some evidence that the inheritance of the narcoleptic syndrome is dependent on a single dominant gene (Baraitser and Parkes, 1978), although narcolepsy has been reported in monozygous twins with both concordance and discordance (Imlah, 1961; Mitchell and Cummins, 1965). Overall, relatives of narcolepsy index cases have at least a 60-fold greater risk of having the disease than do members of the general population. As yet there is no known way of predicting the eventual development of narcolepsy in susceptible individuals. However, Carskadon et al. (1979) recently reported the daughter of a mother with narcolepsy, who developed early onset REM activity for the first time at the age of 14 but who did not have any complaint of sleep disorder.

Initial Features

The first symptom of the narcoleptic syndrome is usually excessive daytime sleepiness, followed within 1–2 years by cataplexy; very occasionally accessory symptoms may antedate the appearance of narcolepsy by as much as 20 years. Daytime sleep is often first noticed at school or during adolescence and it is uncommon for narcolepsy to first present in persons over the age of 40 years. Once established, both narcolepsy and cataplexy are lifelong and do not remit, although symptoms sometimes diminish in frequency or severity for brief periods. Life span is normal.

Wolfenden (1969) found that only 70% of patients with the narcoleptic syndrome had cataplexy as well as narcolepsy, 24% had sleep paralysis and 30% had hypnagogic hallucinations. Only 30% had all four symptoms. Of 190 patients described by Bowling and Richards (1961) and Sours (1963), only 10% had the full tetrad, sleep attacks and cataplexy occurred in 70%, and sleep paralysis alone occurred in less than 5%.

Narcolepsy

Irresistible sleep attacks frequently lead to nicknames at school and subsequently to loss of employment, social disaster or both. Many patients with narcolepsy carry a newspaper cutting giving lurid details of an alleged sufferer. Patients may have from 1 to 10 or, rarely, more sleep attacks daily, most of which last about 30 minutes but occasionally longer. The most common antecedents are boredom and monotony, comfort and warmth. All patients with narcolepsy go to sleep whilst traveling and after eating but also during unusual circumstances such as whilst standing, talking, during intercourse or in the middle of a row. The onset of sleep is sometimes but not always preceded by a feeling of tension, tiredness or warmth and occasionally by a noise or flash in the head. Some but not all people with narcolepsy complain of constant tiredness and attacks are often described as irresistible. If sleep is prevented, patients often feel irritable and may complain of limb ataxia.

Narcolepsy mostly occurs in the afternoon or evening and at home rather than at work. Many patients plan their day around brief, therapeutic naps. Recovery is usually spontaneous or due to noise or other external stimuli. On waking, subjects often feel refreshed, but this finding is probably not of any diagnostic significance in separating normal from abnormal sleep habits (Parkes et al., 1975).

Driving and Narcolepsy

Road traffic accidents are common in people with narcolepsy. Kennedy from the University of Wales in 1929 reported a motor car driver who had sleepy attacks with no warning and periodic double vision lasting 5–10 minutes. Bartels and Kusakcioglu in 1965 reported that 40% of narcoleptics had fallen asleep whilst driving compared with 7% of controls. Despite the high incidence of road traffic accidents, narcolepsy does not constitute an absolute bar to driving in the United Kingdom. Lord Chief Justice Goddard ruled that it would be impossible as well as disastrous to hold that falling asleep at the wheel was any defense to the charge of dangerous driving (1970). If a driver finds that he is getting sleepy, then he must pull his car off the road and stop. Driving ability in a narcoleptic subject probably depends on the frequency, unexpectedness and severity of the attacks, the degree of probability that they might occur whilst driving and the effectiveness of drug control.

Night Sleep

Over 90% of narcoleptics have disordered night sleep, with extreme restlessness and frequent awakenings; accounts of teeth grinding, muscle jerking and body vibration are common. Muscle aching before or after sleep occurs in some patients. The frequency of sleep apnea in narcoleptics is similar to that in normal controls.

Automatic Behavior

Approximately 25–50% of all subjects with narcolepsy have periods of automatic behavior during the day, when they are only half awake. Their behavior is apparently involuntary, with subsequent complete or partial retrograde amnesia, sometimes with loss of any sense of time and occasionally with dysarthric or dysphasic phenomena. The patient may appear drowsy, absent minded or drunk and may produce an apparently meaningless jumble of words. Simple repetitive tasks in familiar surroundings can be performed, but not complex or new demanding tasks. Thus some subjects may carry on an apparently intelligent conversation, drive a car, dial the telephone or transcribe figures at work; others show inappropriate behavior, fail complex tasks or travel to inappropriate destinations (Guilleminault et al., 1975). This type of behavior in narcoleptics is closely similar to that occurring during an attack of transient global amnesia, during sleepwalking or under hypnosis. The pathophysiology is unknown.

Cataplexy

In contrast to narcolepsy which usually results from monotony, cataplexy most often is due to a sudden increase in arousal. The most common precipitants of cataplexy are laughter and surprise. Many sporting activities, e.g., hunting, fishing, playing tennis, cricket or even bowls, are also frequent causes. Cataplexy is most easily provoked when the patient is tired or relaxed and can sometimes be prevented by intense concentration and muscle contraction. Famous cataplectics in American, French and English literature include a priest unable to celebrate mass, a railway signaller paralysed on the approach of a train and a surgeon with attacks triggered by the spurt of blood. David Livingstone, when frightened by the lion, and Silas Marner, when amazed by the sudden appearance of a child, were both motionless but not atonic, with fright or surprise. At a more mundane level, most attacks of cataplexy result from the sight of an unexpected friend or relative, troublesome children or television comedians.

Most attacks of cataplexy are brief and last only seconds and occur without complete loss of motor control, although severe attacks may last several minutes and may be accompanied by total paralysis of voluntary movement with resultant falls and self-injury. This is particularly common following sudden withdrawal of treatment for cataplexy with clomipramine. During an attack of cataplexy, as in periodic paralysis, muscle tone is abolished, the tendon reflexes disappear and the plantar responses may be extensor (Wilson, 1928). The eyes roll or may diverge, the eyelids partially close, the mouth opens, and the facial muscles flicker. Occasionally attacks are unilateral. Recovery of normal motor tone and power is usually rapid. During most attacks of cataplexy the patient is fully alert and with normal sensation (Parkes et al., 1974).

Sleep Paralysis

Sleep paralysis has a close relationship to cataplexy, differing only in time of occurrence and the absence of a trigger mechanism. In both conditions there is paralysis of voluntary movement accompanied by loss of muscle tone and areflexia. In most patients with the narcoleptic syndrome, sleep paralysis is an infrequent occurrence although some subjects have several attacks each night. A characteristic feature, tightness of the chest, constriction or suffocation may result from partial respiratory paralysis. Sleep paralysis, sometimes accompanied by vivid hallucinosis, usually lasts for a few minutes, although characteristically patients cannot estimate the duration of paralysis. A prominent feature is sometimes terror and, to avoid an attack of sleep paralysis, patients may develop complex rituals, request light and noise throughout sleep, and may even request that their wrists be cut after death to escape the fearful possibility of live burial. Recovery from sleep paralysis is usually rapid. Some patients are roused by noise or touch and others can overcome paralysis by an intense effort.

Hypnagogic Hallucinations

As well as occurring on falling asleep or first waking, vivid dreams may also occur in the daytime in people with narcolepsy. This may lead to a consideration of the diagnosis of schizophrenia. Roth and Bruhova (1967), describing the dreams of 451 patients with a number of sleep disorders, considered that visual or auditory hallucinations in narcoleptics were often especially vivid or terrifying, although the subjective nature of dreams in narcoleptics is usually unremarkable.

Epilepsy

Epilepsy has been considered to be part of the narcoleptic syndrome by several authors (Comelade, et al., 1961; Rabending and Schmidt, 1961), largely based on the frequency and reproducibility of attack, loss of muscle tone and facial muscle flickering in cataplexy and also daytime hallucinosis, all features which may occur independently in people with epilepsy. The occasional response of cataplexy to the anticonvulsant drug clonazepam may also suggest a similarity of mechanisms. However, the diagnosis, prognosis and treatment of epilepsy and narcolepsy are different, and narcolepsy should not be considered as an equivalent of epilepsy. There is no evidence that the frequency of epilepsy in narcoleptics is any different from that in the general population.

PSYCHIATRIC ASPECTS OF NARCOLEPSY

Many people with narcolepsy and cataplexy deliberately arrange their lives in order either to diminish the number of attacks of narcolepsy by being active, gambling, joining clubs, arguing or to diminish the number of cataplectic attacks by avoiding hearty laughter, anger, orgasm and family and interpersonal conflict (Parkes and Roy, 1974). A psychogenic basis for narcolepsy (using sleep as an escape from anger, resentment, guilt or sexual impulses) has often been considered, but the only convincing psychotic features in these patients result from hypnagogic hallucinations. Otherwise, most reports of psychosis in narcolepsy are probably due to unrecognized amphetamine psychosis. Psychosis is no more frequent in patients with narcolepsy than would be expected by chance (Braffos and Eltinger, 1963).

The mean I.Q. of narcoleptics has been found to lie within the normal range (Roy, 1976) and personality traits are also usually normal; although, as with epilepsy, distorted self-image, social withdrawal, exclusion by peer groups, difficulty in maintaining employment and heterosexual contacts may lead to the development of a personality disorder (Roy, 1976). However, individual ways of coping and adapting to disability are usually appropriate and, although patients may become discouraged, real attacks of depression are exceptional (Daniels, 1934).

DIFFERENTIAL DIAGNOSIS

The clinical diagnosis of the narcoleptic syndrome depends on a history of narcolepsy and either cataplexy or sleep paralysis in the absence of any evidence of organic brain disease. Narcolepsy may be separated from the one extreme of normal awareness and the other extreme of drowsiness by both the frequency of attack and the unusual surroundings in which day sleep occurs. A family history of similar disability may form useful confirmation of the diagnosis. Cataplexy needs to be distinguished from epilepsy and other causes of drop attacks and, occasionally, also from periodic paralysis or muscle disorder. Automatic behavior very occasionally is the presenting feature of the narcoleptic syndrome and can lead to confusion in diagnosis. Minor manifestations of narcolepsy and cataplexy, including disturbed night sleep, myotonic twitching, trembling, paresthesias as a prelude to sleep spells or loss of muscle tone, hypoglycemia (accompanying amphetamine treatment) and double vision (accompanying cataplexy), may sometimes confuse the diagnosis (Table 4.4).

EEG studies may confirm the diagnosis of narcolepsy and cataplexy and demonstrate REM activity at sleep onset or within 10 minutes of falling asleep. However, it may be necessary to do serial recordings, and a single negative EEG recording (often done under unsatisfactory conditions) does not exclude the diagnosis of the narcoleptic syndrome. Recently 24-hour ambulatory recordings have been shown to be reliable in demonstrating daytime sleep attacks, with REM or nonREM sleep onset (Mounaimne and Riley, 1981).

Table 4.4
Differential Diagnosis of Narcolepsy, Cataplexy, Sleep Paralysis and Epilepsy

	Narcolepsy	Cataplexy	Sleep Paralysis	Epilepsy
Start of attack	Boredom Monotony	Laughter Emotion Sport	Commencement or end of sleep	Unpredictable, may occur in sleep
Usual duration	5–60 minutes	2 seconds–2 minutes	1–3 minutes	5 seconds–15 minutes
Motor symptoms	None	Atonia Areflexia	As cataplexy	Myoclonus Tonic-clonic fits
Awareness	Lost	Retained	Initially retained	Usually impaired
Recovery	Rapid	Immediate	Immediate	Gradual
EEG	Normal sleep or early onset REM	Awake—REM	Awake—Asleep	Specific abnormality

Table 4.5
Differential Diagnosis of Primary Sleep Disorders and Sleep Apnea

	Narcolepsy Alone	Narcoleptic Syndrome	Hypersomnolence	Sleep Apnea
Day sleep	Day sleep attacks	Day sleep attacks	Constant tiredness	Automatic behavior, narcolepsy
Night sleep	Interrupted	Poor, restless, frequent wakenings	Deep, no awakenings, difficult arousal	Restlessness, snoring
Associated features	Nil	Cataplexy, sleep paralysis, hypnagogic hallucinations	Headache, migraine, fainting	Central or respiratory disorder
Sleep onset REM	Present	Present	Absent	Absent
Familial history	Occasional	Frequent	Occasional	Usually nil

DISORDERS OF EXCESSIVE SLEEP

One major difficulty in clinical diagnosis is to distinguish narcolepsy alone and hypersomnolence from the narcoleptic syndrome and from other sleep disorders (Table 4.5).

Sleep Apnea

The diagnosis of hypersomnia-sleep apnea syndrome can usually be made by the history of at least 30 apneas, lasting at least 10 seconds and occurring during 7 hours of sleep. Patients snore and are very restless, with frequent night awakenings and daytime drowsiness. The most common type of sleep apnea is obstructive in origin, and a thick, short neck, obvious mandibular deformity, nasal septal deviation, micrognathia or adenotonsilar enlargement is common. Some patients give a history of operative procedures in the region of the upper respiratory tract. In contrast to obstructive sleep apnea, central sleep apnea is uncommon; in one series, only 2% of all apnea recorded during nocturnal sleep was exclusively central in origin.

Sleep apnea occasionally is associated with the accessory symptoms of the narcoleptic syndrome as well as with narcolepsy. There are reports of sleep paralysis in association with central sleep apnea and of cataplexy with obstructive sleep apnea.

Treatment of sleep apnea is often unsatisfactory, although removal of respiratory obstruction and sometimes weight restriction may be successful. Permanent tracheostomy may effect a cure, although usually at the expense of frequent and serious complications. Protryptiline occasionally may cause slight but definite improvement.

Non-REM Narcolepsy

A distinction has been made between REM and non-REM narcolepsy, the latter condition occurring without accessory symptoms and with persistent hypersomnolence rather than narcolepsy. However, this clinical distinction is not always obvious. Narcolepsy alone may present many years before the appearance of other accessory symptoms, and the age at which early onset REM activity first appears in the narcoleptic syndrome is not known.

Metabolic Disease

Cerebral, metabolic and psychiatric diseases may result in hypersomnia, but these conditions usually present little diagnostic difficulty. Sleep excess or sleep reversal with organic pathology rarely resembles the periodic drowsiness of Gelineau's syndrome, which remains unique and is not associated with structural lesions or induced by drugs.

Sleep Reversal

Mild or extreme degrees of sleep reversal are uncommon but may occur on a genetic basis or with a physiological, psychological or pathological basis. Evidence for a structural lesion is often lacking and the EEG findings are usually normal. No treatment is of avail in this uncommon but distressing condition.

TREATMENT

d-Amphetamine 10–60 mg daily, l-amphetamine 10–80 mg daily, methylphenidate 20–120 mg daily and various other phenylethylamine derivatives have been used for 50 years to treat narcolepsy. None of these is entirely satisfactory and all will cause central stimulation, agitation, anxiety, euphoria and disinhibition as well as frequent peripheral sympathomimetic side effects, in particular tachycardia and sweating (Parkes, 1978). Amphetamine abuse or physical dependence is uncommon in narcoleptics, in whom sudden withdrawal is associated with severe drowsiness lasting a few days but no other serious symptoms. However, there is no doubt that the general availability of these drugs constitutes a threat to public health. In the absence of more satisfactory alternatives, amphetamines should be available by restricted prescription to narcoleptics.

Approximately a third of patients become tolerant to the action of d-amphetamine over 4–8 weeks of treatment, but sensitivity can usually be restored by a brief period of drug withdrawal. Progressive increase in d-amphetamine dosage is usually self-defeating and results in a high incidence of psychosis or sympathomimetic side effects, without any worthwhile increase in alertness. Methylphenidate or the nonphenylethylamine appetite suppressant drug, mazindol 2–8 mg daily, caffeine or ephedrine are sometimes satisfactory alternatives (Parkes and Schachter, 1979). Patients with hypersomnia rather than REM narcolepsy may not be alerted by amphetamines. The excretion of amphetamine is dependent largely upon urinary pH, although attempts to increase central stimulant effects by making the urine alkaline have not been successful.

Yoss and Daly (1959) considered methylphenidate the drug of choice for the treatment of narcolepsy. It caused good or excellent relief of sleepiness in over three quarters of patients. However, more than half of these had some side effects similar to those with amphetamine. If the degree of disability from narcolepsy merits treatment, one policy is to start this with methylphenidate, mazindol or ephedrine and to reserve d-amphetamine for those with poor response or severe disability. Methylamphetamine 2.5–10 mg orally is one of the most powerful CNS stimulants known, but abuse, psychosis and tolerance are considerable problems and this drug is not generally available.

Amphetamine has little or no effect in cataplexy even though most attacks of cataplexy occur when patients are tired. Imipramine and desmethylimipramine are moderately effective, and clomipramine 10–50 mg daily is a very effective treatment for cataplexy in most patients (Hishikawa et al., 1966). This action of tricyclics seems unrelated to any antidepressant effect and tricyclics have little or no action in sleep attacks. The combination of tricyclics with amphetamine might theoretically lower or raise blood pressure, although reports of adverse reactions are infrequent. A minority of patients with cataplexy develop tolerance to clomipramine or weight increase, alteration in libido and impotence. As an alternative to clomipramine, clonazepam 0.5–1 mg daily may be equally effective (Parkes and Schachter, 1979).

Narcolepsy occurs in both dogs and horses and responds to CNS stimulant drugs. These animals also have cataplexy, which responds to atropine and is made worse by physostigmine. The central action of these drugs is shown by the finding that cataplexy in animals is not altered by neostigmine or scopolamine methyl nitrate, drugs which do not cross the blood-brain barrier.

References

Adie, W.J. Idiopathic narcolepsy: A disease sui generis, with remarks on the mechanism of sleep. *Brain* 49:257–306, 1926.

Aserinsky, E., and Kleitman, N. Regularly occurring periods of eye mobility and concomitant phenomena during sleep. *Science* 118:273–274, 1953.

Association of Sleep Disorders Centers. Diagnostic classification of sleep and arousal disorders. *Sleep* 2:1–137, 1979.

Baraitser, M., and Parkes, J.D. Genetic study of narcoleptic syndrome. *J. Med. Genet.* 15: 254–259, 1978.

Bartels, E.C., and Kusakcioglu, O. Narcolepsy: A possible cause of automobile accidents. *Lahey Clin. Found. Bull.* 14:21–26, 1965.

Bonhoeffer, K. Postencephalitic narcolepsy accompanied by cataplexy. *Wien. Klin. Wochenschr.* 41:479–481, 1928.

Bowling, G., and Richards, N.G. Diagnosis of the narcoleptic syndrome. *Cleve. Clin. Q.* 28: 38–45, 1961.

Braffos, O., and Eltinger, L. Psychotic patients with narcolepsy. *Nord. Psychiatr. Tidsskr.* 17:220–226, 1963.

Carskadon, M.A., Harvey, K., Anders, T., and Dement, W.C. Case report: The development of narcolepsy. *Sleep Res.* 8:174, 1979.

Comelade, P., Cadilhac, J., and Passouant, P. Temporal epilepsy and narcoleptic seizures. *Rev. Neurol.* 104:242–245, 1961.

Daly, D.D., and Yoss, R.E. A family with narcolepsy. *Mayo Clin. Proc.* 34:313–319, 1959.

Daniels, L. Narcolepsy. *Medicine* 13:1, 1934.

De Manaceine. *Sleep: Its Physiology, Pathology, Hygiene and Psychology.* Walter Scott, London, 1897.

Gelardi, J.A.M., and Brown, J.W. Hereditary Cataplexy. *J. Neurol. Neurosurg. Psychiatry* 30:455–457, 1967.

Gelineau, J. De la narcolepsie. *Gazette des Hopitaux (Paris)* 53:626–628, 1880.

Gowers, W. *The Borderland of Epilepsy.* Churchill, London, 1907.

Guilleminault, C., Billiard, M., Montplaisir, J., and Dement, W.C. Altered state of consciousness in disorders of daytime sleepiness. *J. Neurol. Sci.* 26:377–393, 1975.

Henneberg, R. Uber genuine Narkolepsie. *Neurol. Zentrabl. 35:*383, 1916.

Hishikawa, Y., Ida, H., Nakai, K., and Kaneko, Z. Treatment of narcolepsy with imipramine and demethylimipramine. *J. Neurol. Sci. 3:*453–459, 1966.

Hishikawa, Y., Man'no, H. Furuya, E., Koida, H., and Kaneko, Z. The nature of sleep attacks and other symptoms of narcolepsy. *Electroencephalog. Clin. Nerophysiol. 24:*1–10, 1968.

Imlah, N.W. Narcolepsy in identical twins. *J. Neurol. Neurosurg. Psychiatry 24:*158–160, 1961.

Jouvet, M., and Delorme, F. Locus caeruleus et sommeil paradoxal. *C.R. Acad. Sci. 154:* 895–899, 1965.

Kennedy, A.M. A note on narcolepsy. *Br. Med. J. 1:*1112–1113, 1929.

Kessler, S., Guilleminault, C., and Dement W.C. A family study of 50 REM narcoleptics. *Acta Neurol. Scand. 50:*503–512, 1974.

Krabbe, F., and Magnussen, G. Familial narcolepsy. *Acta Psychiatr. Neurol. 17:*149–173, 1942.

Lombard, W.P. *Am. J. Psychol. 1:*1, 1887.

Maury. Des hallucinations hypnagogiques ou des erreurs des sens dans l' etat intermediaire entre la veille et le sommeil. *Ann. Med. Psychol. 11:*26–40, 1848.

Mauthner, G. Pathologie und Physiologie des Schlafes. *Wien. Klin. Wochenschr. 3:*445, 1890.

Mounaimne, M., and Riley, T.L. Prolonged Monitoring with Portable Polysomnograph for Diagnosis of Narcolepsy. American EEG Society Annual Scientific Meeting, Chicago, June 1981.

Nan'no, H., Hishikawa, Y., Koida, H., Takahashi, H., and Kaneko, Z. A neurophysiological study of sleep paralysis in narcoleptic patients. *Electroencephalogr. Clin. Neurophysiol. 28:*382–390, 1970.

Parkes, J.D. Amphetamines and alertness. In *Narcolepsy,* edited by Guilleminault, C., Dement, W.C., and Passouant, P. Spectrum Publications, New York, 1978, p. 643.

Parkes, J.D., Baraitser, M., Marsden, D.C., and Asselman, P. Natural history, symptoms and treatment of the narcoleptic syndrome. *Acta Neurol. Scand. 52:*337–353, 1975.

Parkes, J.D., Fenton, G., Struthers, G., Curzon, G., Kantamaneni, B.D., Buxton, B.H., and Record, C. Narcolepsy and cataplexy: Clinical features, treatment and cerebrospinal fluid findings. *Q. J. Med. 43:*425–436, 1974.

Parkes, J.D., and Marsden, C.D. Narcolepsy. *Br. J. Med. 12:*325–334, 1974.

Parkes, J.D., and Roy, A. Neurologic, psychiatric and biochemical aspects of Gelineau's syndrome. *Trans. Am. Neurol. Assoc. 99:*103–106, 1974.

Parkes, J.D., and Schachter, M. Clomipramine and clonazepam in cataplexy. *Lancet ii:* 1085, 1979.

Parkes, J.D., and Schachter, M. Maxindol in the treatment of narcolepsy. *Acta Neurol. Scand. 60:*250–252, 1979.

Passouant, P. In *Narcolepsy,* edited by Guilleminault, C., Dement, W.C., and Passouant, P. Spectrum Publications, New York, 1976, p.3.

Polh, O. Contribution to the pathology of symptomatic narcolepsy. *Dtsch. Z. Nervenheik. 189:*211–217, 1966.

Rabending, G., and Schmidt, G. Narcolepsy with subclinical spasmodic wave paroxysms in the EEG. *Psychiatric Neurol. Med. Psychol. 13:*456–459, 1961.

Rechtschaffen, A., Wolpert, W., Dement, W., Mitchell, S., and Fischer, C. Nocturnal sleep of narcoleptics. *Electroencephalogr. Clin. Neurophysiol. 15:*599, 1963.

Roth, B., and Bruhova, S. Dreams in narcolepsy hypersomnia and dissociated sleep disorders. *Exp. Med. Surg. 27:*187–209, 1967.

Roy, A. Psychiatric aspects of narcolepsy. *Br. J. Psychiatry 128:*562–565, 1976.

Sours, J.A. Narcolepsy and other disturbances in the sleep-walking rhythm: A study of 115 cases with review of the literature. *J. Nerv. Ment. Dis. 137:*525–542, 1963.

Symonds, C.P. Narcolepsy as a symptom of encephalitis lethargica. *Lancet 11:*1214–1215, 1926.

Takahashi, Y., and Jimbo, M. Polygraphic study of narcoleptic syndrome with special reference to hypnagogic hallucinations and cataplexy. *Folia Psychiatr. Neurol. Jpn. 7* (suppl):343, 1963.

Vogel, G. Studies in psychophysiology of dreams: III. The dream of narcolepsy. *Arch. Gen. Psychiatry 3*:421–428, 1960.

Von Economo, C., and Grippe, C. Encephalitis und encephalitis lethargica. *Wien. Klin. Wochenschr. 32* (suppl):393–396, 1919.

Weir Mitchell, S. Remarks of the effects of Anhelonium Lewinii. *Br. Med. J. 2*:1625–1629, 1896.

Wilson, S.A.K. The narcolepsies. *Brain 51*:63–109, 1928.

Wolfenden, W.H. Narcolepsy. *Bull. Post Grad. Med. Univ. Sydney 25*:64–68, 1969.

Yoss, R.E., and Daly, D.D. Criteria for the diagnosis of the narcoleptic syndrome. *Mayo Clin. Proc. 32*:320–328, 1957.

Yoss, R.E., and Daly, D.D. Treatment of narcolepsy with ritalin. *Neurology 9*:171–173, 1959.

Editorial. Medico-legal: Sleepwalking and guilt. *Br. Med. J. 11*:186, 1970.

Chapter 5 Episodic Behaviors due to Neurologic Disorders other than Epilepsy

MICHAEL P. ALEXANDER, M.D.

This chapter considers the episodic disorders of behavior produced by neurological diseases other than epilepsy. These episodic disorders are a heterogeneous group, and a straightforward scheme of classification does not exist. For some, there are true structural lesions of the nervous system: traumatic brain injury and multiple sclerosis are examples. In some, there are no known structural brain lesions, but the underlying physiological events may be at least partially understood: narcolepsy, migraine and transient global amnesia are examples. In others, neither structural lesions nor proven pathophysiological mechanisms are known: paroxysmal choreoathetosis and alcoholic blackouts are examples.

Certain paroxysmal disorders have been omitted because the emphasis in this text is on episodic behaviors which are or might be confused with epilepsy. Many of these omitted disorders are drug related: recurrent hallucinatory experiences ("flashbacks") from chronic hallucinogenic drug use and recurrent psychotic behavior following phencyclidine (PCP) use are examples of delayed drug effects. Acute dystonia, fluctuating involuntary movements and on-off effect in Parkinson's disease are paroxysmal disturbances due to central dopaminergic imbalance. Nocturnal confusion and agitation (so-called sundowning) are common in many neurological settings, expecially among hospitalized, neurologically impaired elderly people. Many marginally compensated metabolic encephalopathies may be abruptly worsened by endogenous metabolic fluctuations or by effects of exogenous factors as simple as meals or medication. There are several uncommon sensory phenomena which are paroxysmal: tic douloureux, various types of tabetic crises, intermittent claudication of the spinal cord, and the many nonepileptic sensory hallucinations and illusions which occur after brain injury (palinopsia, sensory perseverations, thalamic "dazzle," and fluctuating central pain syndromes are but a few examples).

The disorders which are included in this chapter are listed in Table 5.1. They are grouped according to the nature of the primary paroxysmal symptom or sign. Diagnostic confusion with epilepsy seems to occur in 3 major clinical settings: episodic amnesia, episodic confusional states and episodic uncontrollable movements. There will be brief consideration of related fixed neurological disorders, where useful in clarifying pathophysiology of paroxysmal behaviors.

EPISODIC AMNESIA

Transient Global Amnesia

Transient global amnesia (TGA) is a well-known, often-reported syndrome. The clinical features were first outlined by Bender in 1956 as a "syndrome of (an) isolated episode of confusion and amnesia." Detailed description of the attack of amnesia was provided by Fisher and Adams in 1964. Those two reports established the issues of importance and of controversy in this disorder. Over 250 cases of TGA have been described in the English language literature since 1956. Few improve upon the clinical description of the two early reports, but considerable progress has been made in other directions. There are actually several etiologies of the syndrome with variable outcomes, and the neuropathology of amnesia is now better understood. This section will review the clinical syndrome, its causes, its prognosis and the probable pathological substrate.

Table 5.1
Episodic Neurologic Disorders Other than Epilepsy

Transient amnesia	*Transient movement disorders*
Transient global amnesia	Paroxysmal choreoathetosis
Automatic behaviors with amnesia in narcolepsy	Paroxysmal attacks in multiple sclerosis
Alcoholic blackouts	*Related fixed neurological disorders*
Fugue states in epilepsy	Irritable apathy with frontal lobe injury
Transient confusion	Confusional state with right hemisphere stroke
Migraine	Agitated confusion with bilateral limbic infarction
Acute intermittent porphyria	Interictal aggressivity in temporal lobe epilepsy

In the first report, Bender outlined the essential features. This description of the typical attack has not been significantly altered by subsequent reports, but his conclusions about prognosis and lasting residua have been revised. The patients are middle-aged or elderly (average age 60.5, range 41–92). In the attack, the patient becomes suddenly disoriented, agitated or inappropriate; it quickly is clear that a severe memory loss has occurred. The patient may repeat questions about his/her condition or circumstances. Concern and bewilderment are usually prominent. Examination typically reveals no abnormalities other than a severe memory disturbance. The patient is unable to form new memories (anterograde amnesia) and has a loss of memory for events preceding the attack (retrograde amnesia). The latter may sometimes span weeks or years. Other cognitive functions are conspicuously uninvolved. After a few hours, improvement begins. The retrograde amnesia shrinks and some active memory function can be demonstrated. Within several hours the attack is over. The anterograde amnesia is completely resolved, and the retrograde amnesia is brief (minutes to hours); the total amnesic gap is the length of the attack plus the residual retrograde amnesia. There is no postictal depressed neurological function. Bender initially concluded that such attacks never recurred, that there were no observed amnestic or behavioral sequelae and that neurological evaluation was unrewarding.

As additional cases have been reported, many exceptions to the typical sequence have been recognized. Poser and Ziegler (1960) described patients who had several attacks, and in subsequent case reports and series about 25% of patients have had more than 1 attack. Duration of follow-up is obviously significant in determinations of recurrence. A few patients have mild abnormalities on examination during or shortly after the attack; visual field disturbance and mild hemiparesis with reflex asymmetry have been reported.

The etiology of this syndrome has been a source of controversy. Early reports focused on the features of these attacks which were similar or dissimilar to epilepsy or vascular disease. Some early reports stressed the difference between TGA and hysteria. Careful histories have rarely supported the possibility of antecedent head injury (unrecalled) or intoxications. Poser and Ziegler believed posterior circulation ischemia, either atherosclerotic or migrainous, was the likely etiology. Fisher and Adams (1964) weighed the evidence for temporal lobe epilepsy and for vascular disease. The brevity, reversibility, and amnesia supported epilepsy; the age-group did not. The existence of similar patients with permanent amnesia following stroke supported vascular disease. The age of the patients and the high incidence of stroke risk factors and coincident cerebrovascular disease also supported a vascular basis. That

TGA was never seen as a prelude to stroke and that other posterior circulation symptoms and signs were not seen argued against vascular lesions.

Much of the subsequent literature focuses on the issue of etiology. As mentioned above there is no evidence that minor head injuries or alcohol intoxications are pertinent in this syndrome. The striking and dense memory loss combined with a behavioral change may have suggested an hysterical illness, but the differences between TGA and hysterical amnesias are numerous. Hysterical or motivated amnesias usually have the following characteristics which differentiate them from TGA: 1) Hysterical amnesias are often precipitated by a threatening situation; 2) The onset is unrecognized; 3) The patient is found wandering or seeks help in conventional locations (e.g., police); 4) He/she is calm; 5) He/she claims amnesia for much or all personal information but may retain considerable nonpersonal information (e.g., doesn't remember where he/she lives but knows how to get to that town on the rapid transit system); 6) When memory returns, it is sudden. Evans (1966) outlines nicely the differentiation of hysterical amnesia from neurological disorders.

Fisher and Adams (1964) emphasized the possible role of epilepsy in TGA. EEGs obtained after the episode were abnormal in 38% of cases, but no specific pattern was observed. Subsequently, considerable EEG data have been accumulated, almost all of it reflecting EEGs obtained after the TGA had cleared. The most common EEG pattern is a normal background with irregular sharp slowing in the temporal regions, more prominent on the left. Temporal spikes have been described. Several of the published tracings (Rowan and Protass, 1979; Greene and Bennett, 1974: Steinmetz and Vroom, 1972) resemble benign epileptiform transients of sleep (White et al., 1977) and may be of dubious importance. Tharp (1969) recorded an EEG during an attack. The tracing had bilateral paroxysmal temporal sharp activity; no clinical seizure manifestations were observed during the recording. Patients with TGA and a prior history of epilepsy may be selectively excluded from TGA surveys, but a history of epilepsy was noted in fewer than 1% of the cases in the literature. The age at onset, the near universal absence of other complex-partial phenomena and the maintenance of normal attention, language and directed behavior all make epilepsy a very unlikely cause of most cases of TGA. Isolated cases occurring with tumors may be a subgroup of TGA in which epilepsy is relevant.

The evidence for vascular disease is much stronger. There are cases in which typical TGA occurred with a partial visual field defect (Lou, 1968). There are cases in which an unequivocal systemic embolic disorder exists and multiple attacks occur (Steinmetz and Vroom, 1972).

Shuttleworth and Wise (1973) described 2 cases abruptly precipitated by flushing an obstructed intraaortic catheter. Two larger series (Heathfield et al., 1973; Mathew and Meyer, 1974) document the common association with other symptoms of vertebrobasilar insufficiency. Mathew and Meyer (1974) fully evaluated 14 cases of TGA for evidence of vascular disease. Brain scan, electroencephalography, regional cerebral blood flow and four-vessel arteriography all supported the importance of posterior cerebral distribution ischemia. Furthermore, a permanent global amnestic state may occur abruptly after several TGA episodes (Steinmetz and Vroom, 1972) or may occur without preceding TGA (Benson et al., 1974; DeJong et al., 1969). Most reported cases of a permanent amnestic state caused by posterior circulation stroke had clear evidence of bilateral visual field deficits (Benson et al., 1974; Victor et al., 1961), but there are important exceptions. Steinmetz and Vroom (1972) described a patient who reported loss of vision at the outset but who had normal fields when examined. DeJong and others (1969) reported a man with TGA who had bilateral hippocampal lesions at autopsy but no recognized field deficit in life. Four of the cases of Benson et al. (1974) had evidence of only left posterior infarction. The patient of Geschwind and Fusillo (1966) had only left posterior cerebral artery territory infarction; the amnesia slowly resolved over a 3-month period. These cases of permanent "amnestic stroke" provide evidence for a potential substrate of TGA: either bilateral ischemia or left-sided ischemia in the distribution of posterior cerebral artery.

In total, the evidence supporting a primary vascular etiology for TGA seems strong. The circulation involved is probably that of the left lateral posterior choroidal artery. The mechanism is clearly embolic in some cases, but small vessel disease and hemodynamic factors may be pertinent in other cases. Vascular changes in migraine may be relevant in some cases, and related behavioral phenomena in migraine are reviewed in a later section.

There are, however, other documented causes of TGA of which clinicians must remain aware. Hartley et al. (1974) described a patient with an episode of amnesia in whom a large intracranial tumor (pituitary adenoma) compressed the third ventricle and the left medial temporal lobe, thus providing two possible anatomical lesions to cause the amnesia. Three subsequent cases of intracerebral tumor have been reported (Boudin et al., 1975; Lisak and Zimmerman, 1975; Shuping et al., 1980): two with left medial temporal gliomas, the third with a bilateral limbic lesion. The 2 patients with unilateral lesions had normal memory function after the TGA event. Each had suffered a single seizure unrelated to TGA, and in 1 patient there was arteriographic evidence of displacement of the left posterior choroidal artery (Shuping et al., 1980).

Initial EEG was normal in these cases. Either a seizure disorder or localized ischemia might underlie the transient episodes. Both patients developed fixed memory deficits in the subsequent months.

In addition to these unusual cases of intracranial tumors causing TGA, there are scattered reports of drugs producing a similar episode of amnesia. Gilbert and Benson (1972) reported a case of TGA apparently caused by diazepam overdose. Only a diffusely slow EEG with excessive beta activity initially indicated a medication effect. Mumenthaler and others (1979) described 5 cases of TGA following the ingestion of halogenated hydroxyquinolines for diarrhea. Their patients had a longer duration of amnesia, 24–48 hours, and were somnolent, confused and apathetic, unlike typical cases of TGA. The authors cite data from animal research suggesting hippocampal and amygdaloid damage with these drugs. In one other case of TGA related to medication, the mechanism seems basically hemodynamic because of arrhythmias and decreased cardiac output due to digitalis excess (Greenlee et al., 1975). No definite primary effect on memory systems can be attributed to digitalis.

The long-term outcome of TGA has also been controversial. Early reports stressed the infrequency of recurrence and the rarity of lasting stroke in such patients. Subsequently, two general views have emerged. Some long-term follow-up series (Nausieda and Sherman, 1979; Shuping et al., 1980) emphasize the benign outcome: multiple attacks in about 20%, but additional cerebrovascular episodes in only 5%. Other reports have emphasized the possibility of a bleaker outcome (Steinmetz and Vroom, 1972; Mathew and Meyer, 1974). While it is possible that these cases attract medical attention because of poorer outcome, they do provide documentation of unfavorable course: multiple episodes with progressive residual memory disorder, a sudden major amnestic stroke, or a stepwise development of dementia. Recent detailed investigation of neuropsychological residual in ostensibly recovered TGA patients suggests that even fully recovered patients with TGA have permanent, subtle impairment in verbal memory function (Mazzuchi et al., 1980).

Some data are available on the nature of the memory impairment in TGA. Only a few patients have been examined during an attack and even fewer have been rigorously evaluated in the brief time available. Shuttlesworth and Wise (1973) demonstrated that the memory deficit encompassed all sensory modalities. Gordon and Marin (1979) further delineated the deficit in memory, describing failure to recall rhythms or movements. In addition, no manipulation of the learning process (cues, chunking, developing associations) facilitated recall. This profound anterograde amnesia is similar to that seen in alcoholic Korsakoff's disease (Victor et al., 1971), bilateral medial temporal vascular lesions

(Benson et al., 1974) or bilateral medial temporal ablations (Milner et al., 1968). In all cases there seems to be a failure of memory encoding and there is specific evidence from one well-studied patient that the memory problem is in consolidation rather than retrieval functions (Ponsford and Donnan, 1980). The striking retrograde amnesia (of several years in some cases of TGA during the attack) must, however, be interpreted as a failure in retrieval, the neuropsychological mechanism of which is unknown.

The management of a case of TGA must depend upon the physician's perception of the prognostic implications of the disorder. One approach would be the following: 1) a medical evaluation to eliminate polycythemia or potentially embolizing cardiac lesions, e.g., mitral valve prolapse (Shuping et al., 1980); 2) an EEG as a screen for epilepsy as well as drug intoxication; 3) a computed tomography (CT) scan to reveal posterior cerebral artery distribution infarction (amnestic stroke) or medial temporal neoplasm. If a treatable systemic process is not identified and the episode is an isolated one, the patient should be reassured and no further intervention considered. If repeated attacks occur and the EEG reveals epileptiform activity, a trial of antiepileptic medication might be considered. The use of anticoagulation to treat the syndrome may be theoretically unsound (Shuping et al., 1980), but antiplatelet aggregation agents may be useful for repeated attacks, because of the persuasive evidence for a vascular origin of the disturbance.

Neutral State Syndrome: Amnesia and Automatism in Sleep Disorder

Narcolepsy and related disorders are discussed elsewhere in this book. This section will only briefly review one aspect of the idiopathic sleep disorders which may be confused with complex partial seizures: the "neutral state syndrome," automatic behavior in disorders of daytime sleepiness (Guilleminault et al., 1975a; Guilleminault et al., 1975b). In addition to the better known characteristics of narcolepsy and the sleep-apnea syndrome, many persons with excessive daytime somnolence (EDS) have episodes of more prolonged altered consciousness. Guilleminault and others (1975b) described in some detail the nature of these episodes. They occur in patients with narcolepsy and sleep apnea and in patients with EDS without clinical or electroencephalographic criteria of more familiar sleep disorders. The onset is marked by a gradual loss of normal alertness as the patient struggles to remain awake. During an ensuing period of amnesia the patient may continue in his/her activities, with little disturbance of performance in simple tasks. If the activity requires much skill, then deterioration may be noted. Little adaptability of behavior is possible during the spell should sudden changes in activity be needed. Verbal expression is commonly restricted to simple responses. At the end of the episode the patient may not realize how much time has passed, may be amnesic for the interval (although some brief windows of alertness may be recalled), has no postictal impairment, and may discover to his/her embarrassment how he/she passed the time. Guilleminault et al. (1975a) described some colorful examples of distressing automatic behavior. Many of the attacks occur while driving an automobile, with the patient arriving many miles from the intended destination. Such episodes occur in about 60% of narcolepsy patients (Guilleminault et al., 1975a). While we see (or recognize) relatively few patients with sleep disorders, directed questioning has usually uncovered several such episodes in patients with narcolepsy. In our small experience, "neutral state" episodes have been much less common in the sleep-apnea syndrome.

Regardless of primary diagnosis, the electroencephalographic correlate of the automatic behaviors with amnesia is periodic breakthrough of "microsleep." Prolonged EEG monitoring reveals clusters of "microsleep" defined as a brief burst of typical stage I sleep or of central synchronous theta rhythms. During these clusters of microsleep bursts, vigilance and concentration are impaired. When episodes of automatic behavior occur in the context of narcolepsy or sleep apnea, the treatment of the primary disorder is followed. In the smaller number of patients with no other identifiable sleep disorder, no effective treatment has been identified. Antiepileptic medications seem uniformly to worsen the disorder, emphasizing the importance of its recognition.

Alcoholic Blackouts

Alcoholic "blackouts" are episodes of amnesia lasting a limited time during a period of heavy drinking, without loss of consciousness or change in external behavior to betray an ongoing amnesic period. It is our opinion from an informal survey of chronic alcohol abusers that this phenomenon is quite common. Little objective study of the disorder has been undertaken, presumably in part because of the necessity of depending on retrospective reports from a group of generally unreliable historians. Goodwin et al. (1969a and b), in a methodical search, found that 64 of 100 alcoholic subjects had experienced blackouts.

The studies of Goodwin et al. provide a description of the setting of alcoholic blackouts. They usually occur in a period of heavy drinking in a patient who is a confirmed and physically dependent alcoholic. A past history of head injury is commonly elicited. The rate of rise and fall in the blood alcohol level may determine the occurrence of the spell. The blackout itself may be abrupt in onset and in resolution, with a fairly complete amnesic period, or it may be partial, with only vague temporal boundaries. Little is known about the nature of the memory deficit, the pattern of onset and termination, or the physiological mechanism of the amnesia. Tamerin et al. (1971) investigated memory function in states of alcohol intoxication and shed some light on the "blackout syndrome." During a 2-week period of continuous intoxication, several interrelated memory effects were noted. Alcohol impaired short-term recall (1–5 minutes) first. Recall of a previous day's activities was impaired if short-term recall had been impaired on the test day. Only some intoxicated subjects had amnesia for the previous day's activities; there was no relationship to any other neurological or behavioral trait.

With careful history-taking, it appears that alcoholics often have one or more blackout episodes. More pertinent, when a patient with evasive or understated history of alcohol abuse complains of an episode of amnesia, the patient should have a medical evaluation focusing on the medical consequences of alcohol abuse. An electroencephalogram is warranted to explore the possibility of seizures, especially of posttraumatic origin. Such patients should usually be hospitalized for purposes of detoxification, observation for delirium tremens, and psychiatric consultation directed toward treatment of alcoholism.

Nonepileptic Fugue States

The term "poriomania" is a relic of turn-of-the-century European neurology, but it remains a useful term as it identifies a group of patients with fugue states who *also* have epilepsy (Kraeplin, 1909). Poriomania specifically denotes prolonged ambulatory episodes in which normally directed behavior occurs without any indication that the patient will be amnesic for that time. The episode apparently ends abruptly, and the patient is amnesic for the entire interval. Often, afflicted subjects travel a considerable distance during the period of amnesia.

In the many reports of this syndrome, there is often an apparent combination with hysterical or psychogenic fugue states (Mayeux et al., 1979; Stengel, 1941 and 1943; Haller, 1957). Several features define this disorder. The patients have complex partial seizures and, when studied, temporal lobe foci on the electroencephalogram. In addition to the seizures, they have episodes of wandering, often preceded by a feeling of depression and urge to flee and always associated with dense amnesia. The patient usually recovers awareness suddenly, finding himself in an unexpected setting (a bus station, a strange city, walking in a park), realizes that he has had an attack and looks for help. Nothing is known of the behavior during the attack, but unlike patients with TGA, these patients do not come to attention because of a disruptive memory loss. External evidence (bus tickets, gas receipts, distance travelled) suggests that behavior during the spell must be fairly normal. Poriomania seems restricted to those temporal lobe epileptics who are also depressed in the interictal period.

These episodes differ from complex partial status epilepticus, in which behavior is clearly abnormal (Mayeux and Lender, 1978) even when initially not recognized as epilepsy (Wells, 1975). Various interpretations of poriomanic episodes have been proffered. They are probably not ictal because of the long duration of the spells and the complex activities apparently completed. They may, however, represent sequential postictal confusional periods (Gastaut et al., 1956) or may be prolonged postictal automatism (Mayeux et al., 1979) as suggested for the famous physician patient of Jackson. Stengel has outlined an excellent argument that poriomania differs little from other types of psychogenic wandering and that these patients all have 3 features in common: 1) severe depression, 2) some personal episode of loss of consciousness (epilepsy, head injury, or alcoholic stupor), and 3) a need to escape from an overwhelming life situation. It is not obvious why these fugue states are more common in epileptic patients with temporal lobe seizures, but the striking premonitory mood swings in our patients suggest the importance of limbic structures. Until a patient is studied during and after an episode, the exact physiological mechanism will remain uncertain.

Some suggestions about management can be offered even in the absence of complete elucidation of pathophysiology. First, a detailed history of predisposing factors for epilepsy (family history, febrile convulsions, history of intracranial infection, head injury) and a methodical survey of possible complex partial symptoms should be undertaken. Electroencephalography should be performed, preferably with sleep deprivation and nasopharyngeal electrodes and, probably, long-term recording. A diagnosis of epilepsy alone demands anticonvulsant treatment. In addition, the patients whom we have seen have had a reduction in wandering episodes with antiepileptic medications (Mayeux et al., 1979). Second, a detailed review of the psychiatric history, alcohol and drug use, vegetative and affective symptoms is required. Many of these patients are depressed and suicide has been reported (Stengel, 1941 and 1943). Proper treatment of depression and follow-up is imperative.

TRANSIENT CONFUSION

Migraine

Migraine headache is a paroxysmal disorder which afflicts as many as 10% of adults and 4% of children (Bille, 1962). When the headache is associated with neurological dysfunction, it is usually referred to as a complicated migraine. There are several relatively common varieties of complicated migraine: hemiplegic migraine with or without aphasia (Riley and Massey, 1980), ophthalmoplegic migraine and hemianopic migraine. The discussion to follow is limited to two varieties of complicated migraine with prominent behavioral components: basilar artery migraine and acute confusional migraine.

Basilar artery migraine was first described in detail by Bickerstaff (1961a and b), but isolated cases were described before this. Since his clinical descriptions, several detailed reports have appeared. Adolescent females are affected most often, but cases have been described in young men and in adults; there are many examples of patients with a long history of more benign migraine who develop symptoms of basilar migraine in later life (Evans, 1966; Swanson, 1978; Lees and Watkins, 1963). A family history of migraine is common. The aura may be any combination of symptoms attributable to deficits of posterior cerebral circulation: teichopsia, unformed visual hallucinations, loss of vision, vertigo, tinnitus, gait ataxia and perioral paresthesias have been the most common. Some surprisingly discrete localized symptoms have been reported: simultaneous paresthesias of the right side of the face and of the left side of the body for instance (Pearce and Foster, 1965).

Bickerstaff originally reported episodes of loss of consciousness in 25% of patients with basilar migraine (1961a and b). Subsequent surveys vary in reported incidence. Preselection for cases with loss of consciousness may cause this variation. Golden and French (1975) found no loss of consciousness in 8 young children with basilar migraine, but Swanson and Vick (1978) described loss of consciousness in 8 of 12 patients of varying age (8–46 years). When consciousness is lost, there is a common clinical pattern. Characteristically, onset of the ictus is gradual, often preceded by a dreamlike state. Although some patients have lost consciousness rapidly and slumped to the ground, most have time to sit down or lie down. Several patients have described the episode as similar to falling asleep. The unconsciousness is not deep; all patients have been at least partially arousable. The loss of consciousness usually occurred at the peak of the aura, was brief in duration (2–30 minutes), terminated suddenly, and was followed by a severe headache.

Other behavioral disturbances have been described in association with basilar migraine. Young children may become agitated or lethargic (Golden and French, 1975). Confusion, feelings of fear and depersonalization, formed (monsters) and unformed (colorful scotomata) visual hallucinations and transient amnesia may also occur at the peak of the aura (Poster and Ziegler, 1960; Evans, 1966; Gilbert and Benson, 1972; Pearce and Foster, 1965). The amnestic episodes are very similar to TGA; only the age of the patient and the history of migraine might help in establishing the etiology. Finally, basilar migraine has culminated in convulsions in some patients. Camfield et al. (1978) described 3 children with seizures (1 focal motor, 1 focal becoming generalized and 1 generalized) occurring at the height of the aura. One additional child had typical basilar migraines in addition to three nocturnal generalized seizures.

The coincidental occurrence of basilar migraine and epilepsy in some patients highlights the controversial relationship between migraine in general and epilepsy. Without attempting to address this larger issue, a few observations about basilar migraine and epilepsy may be useful. In that minority of cases with seizures at the peak of the aura, the routine electroencephalogram has been abnormal with epileptiform activity, either focal temporal discharges or bilateral posterior synchronous discharges (Camfield et al., 1978). In patients with typical basilar migraine (with or without loss of consciousness), randomly obtained EEGs may be abnormal in up to 50% of cases (Hockaday and Whitty, 1969); however, many series have a low incidence of abnormal tracings (Bickerstaff, 1961a and b; Swanson and Vick, 1978; Golden and French, 1975). Of greater interest than random EEGs are those few obtained near or during an attack. Slatter (1968) recorded shortly after an attack in a 46-year-old man who was still confused at the time of the recording. There was generalized, symmetrical delta activity; a repeat recording 1 month later demonstrated normal background with only some minor posterior slowing. Lapkin et al. (1977) captured similar tracings in 2 children within one day of their attacks. The slowing was more clearly occipital, rhythmic and synchronous, but subsequent follow-up tracings were normal. Swanson and Vick (1978) happened to capture the onset and period of unconsciousness in a 23-year-old woman. A normal background was replaced by symmetrical occipital spike and slow wave activity, initially during photic stimulation but eventually sustained beyond the photic stimulus. In summary, the random EEG in patients with basilar artery migraine may be abnormal but in a nonspecific way. An EEG obtained during or very shortly after an attack may be markedly abnormal, typically showing diffuse, symmetrical, posteriorly predominant delta rhythms. A minority of cases are associated with seizures at the peak of the aura. These patients may have epileptiform discharges on EEG, but clinically they behave similarly to the more typical cases.

Altered behavior during basilar migraine may then take several forms. At the crest of the aura, gradual fading of consciousness may occur. Confused wakefulness, arousable stupor or generalized convulsions may be seen. The first two presumably represent ischemia of critical ascending arousal systems in the mesencephalic or diencephalic reticular system; the EEGs obtained during or near attacks support this hypothesis. Convulsions may represent ischemic effects on potentially epileptic brains (Lees and Watkins, 1963) or repeated ischemic migrainous auras (Camfield et al., 1978).

The major differential diagnoses are age dependent. In children, posterior fossa tumors, encephalitis, subarachnoid hemorrhage, and Leigh's syndrome might all be considered until the benign course or repeated attacks make the etiology clear. After a first attack, in a child too young to accurately describe the illness, an evaluation designed to eliminate the above disorders would be indicated: CT scan, lumbar puncture and pyruvate decarboxylase determination. In adults, atherosclerotic vascular disease would be the major differential. Young age at onset or a lifelong history of migraine, a strong family history of migraine and the absence of residual signs would all militate against atherosclerotic vascular disease. However, a first attack of complicated migraine in middle age may force an evaluation of the extracranial vascular system. Many examples of fixed residual deficits have been reported (Pearce and Foster, 1965; Connor, 1962) and, in the absence of conclusive history of migraine, arteriography should be considered.

A separate clinical syndrome of behavioral disorder associated with migraine headaches is acute confusional migraine (ACM). Alterations in alertness and responsiveness during a migraine attack have long been recognized. Lance and Anthony (1966) compiled detailed accounts of migraine attacks in 500 consecutive patients and noted 34 patients who had a history of confusion or disorientation during their headaches. Some of their patients were subsequently amnestic for the period of confusion. The nature of these confusional periods was not further specified except that they occurred in patients with carotid distribution symptoms and in patients with basilar distribution symptoms. No attempt was made to isolate a particular syndrome of migraine with confusion.

Since that tabulation, several small series have confirmed the typical features of acute confusional migraine (Gascon and Barlow, 1970; Emery, 1977; Ehyai and Fenichel, 1978). These reports total 13 patients, all between the ages 5 and 16, with confusional states during migraine attacks. Other reports emphasizing different aspects of the headache also include similar cases which suggest ACM. Golden and French (1975) focused on the posterior circulation elements in their cases, but their case with screaming and irritability is similar to reported ACM cases. Pearce and Foster (1965) stressed the complications of migraine, but confusion occurred in several of their cases. "Confusion" of course is not a specific term and is often not further described but it may misrepresent many other behavioral phenomena such as aphasia, hallucinatory states, lethargy, etc. A few conclusions about confusion occurring during migraine can be made: it is more common in children but definitely may occur in adults; in children it may be the first manifestation of recurrent vascular headaches. Confusion is most typically noted at the peak of the aura, preceding the actual headache. In children, at least, there may be lethargic unresponsiveness, with purposeless movements or an agitated and combative state. The associated clinical symptoms and signs and the electroencephalographic data suggest that confusion may occur in migraines of either carotid system or of the basilar system, but the right carotid and basilar territories seem more frequently represented than is the left carotid system. The period of confusion may last only minutes, typical of a migrainous aura, but most childhood cases have been of longer duration, 3–25 hours. The attack often ends with sleep. Amnesia for the confusional period is common. EEGs at or near the episode have usually shown focal hemispheric slowing, only rarely the bilateral synchronous delta activity of deep, reticular activating system dysfunction.

Diagnosis in the setting of long-standing migraine headaches is not difficult. When occurring as the earliest vascular headaches in a small child who is initially agitated and incoherent and then amnesic, the diagnosis may be more difficult. A family history of migraine is common. The differential diagnosis includes encephalitis, intoxication and epilepsy. EEG, spinal fluid evaluation and a toxic screen may be required if the nature of the episode is not clear.

The cause of confusion in these cases is not known. Involvement of deep midline structures in the posterior circulation may be responsible for some. Simple focal transient ischemia during the vasoconstrictive phase of the migraine seems likely in a few cases in which confusion is brief and occurs at the peak of the aura. For most cases the long duration without permanent residual suggests a period of cerebral edema (Gascon and Barlow, 1970). Two adult syndromes may shed light on the reversible functional disorder in ACM. Infarction in the distribution of the right middle cerebral artery may produce a lasting confusional state in adults (Mesulam et al., 1976). The confusional state is prominent even in cases without hemiparesis. One author of that report has often commented on the rarity of clinically recognized right brain strokes without hemiparesis (Geschwind, personal communication). We have occasionally recognized such patients. They have usually come to medical attention because of confusion, bizarre behaviors, apathy or reduplication.

The second syndrome in adults which may be relevant to ACM is the agitated delirium reported after infarctions in posterior-cerebral artery distribution (Horenstein et al., 1974; Medina et al., 1974). The patients in these reports had severe and lasting agitated confusion following medial and inferior temporal-occipital infarctions, unilateral in either hemisphere or bilateral. The mechanism of this disorder is not clear; the neurological literature is rife with cases with similar lesions reported for their visual agnosia, prosopagnosia or memory disorders, but without this behavior change. These two syndromes in adults suggest possible neuropathological substrates for reversible confusion and agitation in juvenile migraineurs.

Basilar artery migraine and acute confusional migraine have been successfully treated with a variety of agents. Successful prophylaxis of migraine headaches has been achieved with phenobarbitol (Gascon and Barlow, 1970) and ergotamine, dilantin or propanolol (Swanson and Vick, 1978). In the few cases with associated seizures, dilantin (Lapkin et al., 1977) has been effective in headache and seizure prevention. We suspect that any drug with reasonable preventative effectiveness in migraine might be successful in these syndromes.

Acute Intermittent Porphyria

Acute intermittent porphyria (AIP) is one of several related disorders of hepatic heme biosynthesis. The relevance of this hepatic biosynthetic disorder to neurology is twofold: neurological signs and symptoms are common, and a large number of medications prescribed by neurologists can precipitate an acute attack of the disease. The relevance of AIP to this chapter lies in the occasional occurrence of an acute encephalopathy as the primary manifestation of the disease. Many comprehensive reviews of AIP are available (Sergay, 1979; Becker and Kramer, 1977; Stein and Tschudy, 1970; Waldenstrom, 1957), and only a brief summary will be found here.

AIP is an unusual disorder, inherited as an autosomal dominant (Tschudy et al., 1975). It is more common in women (about 60% of cases). Average age at onset is earlier in women (mid 20s) than in men (mid 30s), perhaps reflecting the effects of estrogen (Stein and Tschudy, 1970). There is no unequivocal evidence that affected patients have any specific clinical neurological, psychiatric or endocrine disorder between the acute attacks.

The underlying biosynthetic deficit is a deficiency of the enzyme uroporphyrinogen I synthetase which causes an accumulation of porphobilinogen (PBG) and diminished heme synthesis. Feedback from the decrease in heme leads to an increase in the initial reaction of heme synthesis, the conversion of succinyl-coenzyme A and glycine to δ-aminolevulinic acid (δ-ALA) by ALA-synthetase (ALAS). Between attacks, urinary and blood PBG and ALA are mildly elevated, but during attacks there is an additional dramatic increase (Stein and Tschudy,

1970). The mechanism by which these increases result in neurological dysfunction is uncertain, although a direct effect on neurotransmitter receptors (especially for γ-aminobutyric acid) has been described (Becker and Kramer, 1977). The limited neuropathology, primarily peripheral and central demyelination, is well reviewed by Becker and Kramer (1977).

Transformation from a stable, asymptomatic state with modestly increased δ-ALA and PBG to the symptomatic condition is usually precipitated by factors such as drugs which induce hepatic ALAS activity, steroidal hormones, menstruation, intercurrent infections, or starvation (dieting) (Stein and Tschudy, 1970). Neurologists must be alert to the fact that many common medications might precipitate an attack. These include phenytoin, phenobarbital (and other barbiturates), primidone, chlordiazepoxide, amphetamine, ergotamine and imipramine. Sergay (1979) includes a more complete list. The period of latency between drug use and onset of symptoms may be as long as 4 weeks. Prior exposure to a drug without complications does not eliminate risk from the same drug on subsequent exposure.

Once an attack commences, all clinical symptoms and signs are produced through different levels of neurological impairment (Becker and Kramer, 1977). Autonomic neuropathy occurs in about 95% of cases, the most common manifestations being abdominal pain, vomiting, constipation, ileus, urinary retention, tachycardia, hypertension or *hypotension*, and sweating abnormalities. Severe autonomic instability is one of the causes of death in an acute attack. The initial symptom in 75% of cases is abdominal pain, and there is evidence of a sensorimotor peripheral neuropathy in half of the cases—motor impairment is typically more severe than sensory loss (Sergay, 1979). An ascending pattern may suggest Guillain-Barre syndrome. Unlike in Guillain-Barre syndrome, cranial nerves may be involved. Rapid progression to total quadriparesis, bulbar paresis and respiratory failure is a not uncommon outcome, the other route to a fatal outcome in AIP. Peripheral neuropathy is seldom the initial manifestation of an attack, however.

AIP is relevant to this chapter because it also produces central nervous system dysfunction which may recur with each attack. In the many large reviews of AIP, alteration in mental status is reported in about 30% of cases. Unlike peripheral neuropathy these symptoms may be the initial features of the disease, and, if not the *first* symptoms, they are often the dominant ones. Unfortunately, these behavioral changes are seldom reported in detail. Patients are described as confused, hallucinating, lethargic, depressed, anxious, psychotic, deranged and hysterical. From these various descriptions, it seems that an acute confusional state with hallucinations is the most common mental disorder.

Most patients described as psychotic are probably also in this agitated confusional state. Lethargy progressing to coma is occasionally seen. Some patients apparently do seem to suffer from anxiety or depression, while remaining relatively free of evidence of confusion. Some remain depressed after complete resolution of the acute attack (Stein and Tschudy, 1970); it is not known if this is on the basis of residual CNS impairment. An additional important form of recurrent CNS involvement in AIP is epilepsy. Convulsions (almost invariably generalized time clonic seizures) occur eventually in the course of an acute attack in about 10–20% of cases (Waldenstrom, 1957; Goldberg, 1959) and may occasionally be the presenting feature of the disease. The possible consequences of inappropriate anticonvulsant selection in these patients should be obvious. Barbiturate medications worsen the biochemical and clinical features of the disease.

The final neurological manifestation of AIP is neuroendocrine. The syndrome of inappropriate ADH secretion (SIADH) occurs in a small fraction of acute attacks (Stein and Tschudy, 1970), with a dramatic decrease in serum sodium seen occasionally. Abnormalities in serum electrolytes may play a role in the development of convulsions or of encephalopathy, but correction of these abnormalities often produces no change in mental status. When evaluated, inappropriate secretion of growth hormone has also been documented (Stein and Tschudy, 1970).

Diagnosis of AIP is not difficult given the complete clinical picture, but bouts of abdominal pain and/or confusion may resolve spontaneously before the diagnosis is considered; the delay before diagnosis is commonly 6 months or more. The serious neurological sequelae are often iatrogenically produced by symptomatic treatment of abdominal pain or anxiety before the diagnosis is made (Sergay, 1979). With reference to the CNS signs, acute psychotic behavior in a previously normal individual should always trigger a search for a neurological, medical or toxic etiology. The diagnosis may be suggested by a positive Watson-Schwartz test and confirmed by a quantitative determination of urinary ALA or PBG. Routine neurological diagnostic tests between attacks are normal (CSF examination and brain scan) or nonspecifically abnormal; the electroencephalogram may show diffuse slowing, and the electromyogram may show evidence of denervation in the presence of clinical neuropathy (Stein and Tschudy, 1970). Lead intoxication, causing neuropathy and encephalopathy, is the only disorder which should mimic AIP but should cause less paroxysmal features. Urinary ALA is increased in lead intoxication, but coproporphyrin rather than PBG is elevated.

Treatment of AIP is two-pronged. Prevention of attacks is the major goal, assisted by high carbohydrate diet and avoiding precipitant medications. In women whose attacks are associated with menses, oral contraceptives may be helpful. If an attack occurs, treatment consists of several simultaneous measures (Sergay, 1979): 1) correction of metabolic disorders such as hyponatremia, 2) a high glucose intake (400 to 1000 gm/24 hours) and 3) suppression of ALAS with intravenous hematin. Sedation may be achieved safely with chlorpromazine, and seizures treated with diazepam or valproate (Biagini et al., 1979). Autonomic hyperactivity may be reduced by intravenous propanolol.

An unusual disease, AIP demands early recognition of its recurrent autonomic and/or behavioral signs and symptoms. Mortality is high in unrecognized cases and residual disability may be severe. The potential for iatrogenic neurological complication is very high.

TRANSIENT MOVEMENT DISORDERS

Paroxysmal Choreoathetosis

Paroxysmal choreoathetosis is an unusual disorder, although it may be more common than generally recognized. Cases have entered the neurological literature labeled as reflex epilepsy, movement-induced epilepsy, tonic epilepsy, kinesigenic choreoathetosis, nonkinesigenic choreoathetosis, and paroxysmal dyskinesias. The original description belongs to Gowers (1901), who believed the attacks to be epileptic. Mount and Reback (1940) described the nonkinesigenic form of the disorder and proposed that it was intrinsically a movement disorder. Kertesz (1967) and Goodenough et al. (1978) have proposed a classification on clinical criteria which is most helpful in clinical recognition.

The disorders included in this section consist of episodic "short paroxysm(s) of unilateral or generalized tonic, choreiform and athetoid movements and posturing usually precipitated by movement" (Kertesz, 1967). Excellent photographic montages may be found in Kertesz (1967) and Kato and Araki (1969). At the time of the review by Goodenough et al. (1978), 79 cases of idiopathic paroxysmal choreoathetosis (PCA) could be collected and 64 were clearly precipitated by movement (kinesigenic). The onset of PCA in the kinesigenic cases is in childhood or adolescence. Males predominate considerably, and the family history is positive although variably in an autosomal dominant or an autosomal recessive pattern. The onset of PCA in the nonkinesigenic patient is in infancy or very early childhood. Male predominance is not marked. The pattern of inheritance is invariably autosomal dominant.

The attacks consist of the abrupt onset of abnormal involuntary movements. In the kinesigenic group, sudden movement (especially after a quiet period) may induce an attack, followed by a short refractory period. The movements may be unilateral with generalization, symmetrically bilateral or strictly unilateral. Rapid choreoathetoid movements are more common than slower dystonic movements. Duration is brief (less than 2 minutes) but frequency is high. In the nonkinesigenic group, the movements are not precipitated by any special activity; some patients describe sensitivity to alcohol ingestion. The attacks are similar in form to kinesigenic attacks, but they are much more prolonged (minutes to hours) and more infrequent. In both forms, the attacks are commonly preceded by a vague sensory prodrome in those limbs eventually affected by the paroxysm. In both forms the attacks may occasionally be aborted by intentional arrest of all movement or by pressure upon the affected limb. In the kinesigenic disorder, gradual preliminary movement or "warm-up" before rapid movements may forestall attacks. During attacks there is no alteration of consciousness, and afterwards there is no lethargic state or headache.

Between attacks, the neurological examination remains normal. Several paroxysms have occurred during EEG recordings and no paroxysmal EEG patterns accompanied the movement disorder. About 40% of patients have had abnormal interval routine EEGs but no specific patterns have been described, and even the patients with abnormal resting EEGs lack paroxysmal epileptic activity during the bursts of PCA (Goodenough et al., 1978). An abnormal CT scan was reported in one patient, demonstrating brain stem atrophy and enlarged fourth ventricle (Kato and Araki, 1969). Neuropathological examination of 2 cases revealed only slight depigmentation of substantia nigra in 1 case (Stevens, 1980) and of locus ceruleus in the other (Kertesz, 1967).

The pathophysiology of the disorder is unknown. Reflex epilepsy or basal ganglia disease has been suggested by most reports, based upon clinical evidence and supposition; a disorder of the extrapyramidal motor systems seems the more probably cause. The paroxysmal nature of the attacks and favorable clinical response to anticonvulsants, on the other hand, favor an epileptic basis. As there are other extrapyramidal disorders with paroxysmal features (torticollis, early torsion dystonia, on-off phenomena in Parkinson's disease and phenothiazine-induced dystonia are examples) and as anticonvulsants may benefit other paroxysmal nonepileptic disorders (trigeminal neuralgia for instance), the evidence for a primary extrapyramidal disorder is considerably stronger.

The differential diagnosis of PCA includes epilepsy, hypocalcemia with idiopathic hypoparathyroidism, cerebral palsy, paroxysmal attacks in multiple sclerosis and, perhaps, hysteria. There are rare cases of movement-induced epilepsy with abnormal ictal EEGs (Whitty et al., 1964). In addition, epilepsy originating in the supplementary motor cortex may produce contralateral tonic seizures with movements similar to PCA. One such case with movement-induced seizures has been described (Falconer et al., 1963). Routine and ictal EEGs may be required to establish the diagnosis. Idiopathic hypoparathyroidism with typical kinesigenic PCA and basal ganglion calcification has been described (Arden, 1953; and Tabaee-Dadeh et al., 1972). In both patients, PCA stopped with correction of the hypocalcemia. The diagnosis of cerebral palsy with associated PCA is readily made by the abnormal routine neurological examination. Paroxysmal movement disorders in multiple sclerosis (MS) will be described in the next section. A diagnosis of hysteria will surely be applied to these patients only by those ignorant of the existence of PCA. A patient who presents with PCA and a normal neurological examination should have a serum calcium determination, a routine EEG and, if possible, an EEG while an attack is provoked. Routine CT scanning is indicated only for patients with an abnormal examination, an epileptiform EEG or hypocalcemia.

Treatment of the kinesigenic variety of PCA is straightforward. Numerous antiepileptic medications (phenytoin, carbamazepine, primidone, phenobarbitol, and valproic acid) have been reported effective, but phenytoin is the generally preferred drug. Levodopa has been effective in the single patient in whom it has been tried (Loong and Ong, 1973). The nonkinesigenic disorder has been more difficult to treat; anticonvulsants are rarely helpful. There is a recent brief report of 2 patients who responded to haloperidol, 0.5 mg at bedtime (Coulter and Donofrio, 1980). This drug should be the first attempted in the nonkinesigenic variety of PCA. In both forms of PCA the frequency of attacks decreases during adulthood. To avoid potential long-term toxicity of medication, drug withdrawals periodically in adulthood are warranted.

Multiple Sclerosis

While not likely to be confused with epilepsy by the experienced clinician, paroxysmal abnormalities in the initial stages of MS may cause some difficulty in diagnosis. Thus, a brief consideration is worthwhile.

Paroxysmal attacks in MS had been described for many years, but clear descriptions of the common forms of paroxysmal behavior in MS have been available only in the past 20–25 years. Stereotyped, transient disturbances of function occurring repetitively over weeks or months are characteristic of tonic "seizures," spinal sensorimotor "seizures," paroxysmal dysarthria and ataxia, and paroxysmal akinesia. The variations of these attacks are described below, but they all have certain qualities in common.

In any patient the attacks are stereotyped. Paroxysmal attacks which recur later in the disease may be identical to the first bout. There is never any alteration of consciousness. The paroxysmal attacks are abrupt in onset, brief in duration (less than 2 minutes), occur at high frequency (up to several times an hour), usually occur during an active stage of the disease (indeed may qualify as a relapse by themselves), and stop spontaneously. The attacks considered here do not include such fleeting neurologic symptoms as Lhermitte's sign, transient visual impairment after exertion, or extensor or flexor spasms. The paroxysmal disorders may occur early in the disease, when the diagnosis is unclear, or late when the diagnosis is evident. The neurologic examination between attacks may not demonstrate significant disturbance in those functions affected during the attack. Review of several large series of patients with paroxysmal dysfunctions in MS reveals that 5–10% of all patients with MS have paroxysmal attacks.

A transient motor disturbance called "tonic seizures" is one of the common forms of paroxysmal attack. First described by Matthews (1958), several reports document the essential characteristics (Matthews, 1975; Espir and Millac, 1970; Osterman and Westerberg, 1975). They are unilateral and may spare the leg and/or the face. They are preceded by a brief sensory aura on the affected side, but the movements begin very abruptly. Limb postures are variable but tonic arm flexion and leg extension are most common. In a minority of cases the contractions are painful. Rarely, there is simultaneous dysarthria. Tonic seizures may be precipitated by hyperventilation. Joynt and Green (1962) provide photographs of the typical postures. Many examples of these tonic "seizures" have been recorded during EEG monitoring, but none has ever revealed any ictal disturbance.

Paroxysmal dysarthria and ataxia is the other common form of paroxysmal disorder in MS. Andermann and co-workers first clearly described this disturbance in 1959. Again, a brief sensory prodrome of unilateral perioral paresthesias may occur, but in many cases there is simply sudden severe disturbance in articulation associated with unilateral or bilateral limb and trunk ataxia. There is no language disorder. As with tonic "seizures," simultaneous EEG recording has failed to demonstrate any associated epileptiform activity.

Spinal sensorimotor "seizures" are rare (Espir and Millac, 1970; Ekborn et al., 1968) but provide the clearest window to the potential pathophysiology of all paroxysmal attacks. The sudden onset of tonic stiffening in one leg is quickly followed by painful paresthesias in the other leg. Other paroxysmal motor disorders are very rare and remain poorly defined (paroxysmal akinesia, for example).

Paroxysmal sensory symptoms of several types have been reported. Paresthesias, pain and, very rarely, itching have been described (Espir and Millac, 1970; Osterman and Westerberg, 1975). Paresthesias have been in a limited region, very brief and very frequent. Pain has been deep and cramping when associated with tonic seizures but has been sharp and lancinating, in a stereotyped but restricted area, when occurring alone. Trigeminal neuralgia in MS is an example of this latter form.

The mechanism of these attacks is unknown, but spinal sensorimotor "seizures" may provide the best clue. Ekborn et al. (1968) outlined how contiguous demyelinated axous may, by direct contact (ephaptic transmission), give rise to crossed sensory and motor impulses. Similar ephaptic transmission could account for the tonic contractions precipitated by movement. A brain stem lesion would be the source for ephaptic "crosstalk" in paroxysmal dysarthria and ataxia. Osterman and Westerberg (1975) provide cogent reasons for believing that all of the paroxysmal disorders have similar pathophysiology. In a disease of myelin and white matter, the concept of nonsynaptic, ephaptic, transmission between adjacent tracts and pathways is pleasantly unifying. Furthermore, there are two experimental settings in which such axon-to-axon transmission has been demonstrated (Rasminsky, 1978; Seltzer and Devor, 1979).

Another feature which all paroxysmal attacks in MS have in common is a favorable response to certain anticonvulsants, carbemazepine and, to a lesser degree, phenytoin (Espir and Mallac, 1970; Joynt and Green, 1962; Espir and Watkins, 1966; Miley and Forster, 1974). Overall, carbamazepine is clearly preferable. The effect is specific for the paroxysmal symptoms and not generally useful in the basic demyelinating disorder. There are several reports of cases in which ACTH produced improvement in the MS but not the attacks, and where carbamazepine promptly blocked the attacks without affecting the progression of other neurological signs (Miley and Forster, 1974). The effective dose is remarkably low: 100–400 mg each day. When phenytoin has been effective, standard anticonvulsant doses have been used. The attacks eventually remit in all cases, thus, evidence that a relapse is reversing should signal an attempt to discontinue medications.

RELATED FIXED NEUROLOGICAL DISORDERS CAUSING PAROXYSMAL BEHAVIOR

Additional behaviors potentially confused with epilepsy are those unpredictable outbursts found in patients with stable, recognizable brain disease. The most obvious example of this is frontal lobe dysfunction. Patients with extensive frontal lobe disease are often irritable, apathetic and euphoric. The irritability, poor impulse control, poor social judgment and lack of organized remorse all so common in frontal lobe disease predispose these patients to explosive outbursts (Damasio,

1979). These outbursts often arise out of a prevailing apathy and uncon-
cern. They may be triggered by trivial or irrelevant stimuli: a child
letting a door slam, a spouse reluctant to let the patient drive, etc. It
ends quickly, with the patient promptly minimizing the explosion.

We have evaluated and followed many patients at the Neurobehavior
Unit of the Boston Veterans Administration Medical Center who have
these unexpected outbursts after head injury, anoxic injury, frontal
tumors and infarcts. Careful history reveals that these spells have no
aura, and no prodrome is reported. They are not stereotyped; each is
dependent on the situation in which it develops. Depending on the
extent of underlying brain injury, the patient may be able to remember
the entire episode. No convulsive or automatic behaviors are seen. Many
had been started on anticonvulsants to control this problem but without
success. We have had limited success treating these patients with
chronic low dose phenothiazines.

Two other instances of fixed brain lesions which may present as
acute confusional states have already been briefly mentioned in the
context of acute confusional migraine. When the brain lesion is developed and persistent the diagnosis may be clear, but initially it may be
uncertain. Acute right brain strokes without hemiparesis may present
as acute ambulatory confusion (Mesulam et al., 1976). The patients talk
fluently and have no focal neurologic signs. They are agitated and seem
to be hallucinating; coherent conversation is impossible. Diagnosis has
been made by nuclide and CT scanning. The confusion may be permanent. Bilateral posterior limbic infarction may produce acute agitated
delirium (Horenstein et al., 1967; Medina et al., 1974). These patients
characteristically rest quietly unless stimulated; then they become extremely agitated and aggressive. Because the lesions lie in the posterior
cerebral artery territories bilaterally, an amnesic state and various
degrees of cortical blindness are seen. The confusional state is permanent. There is no known successful treatment for either of these confusional states.

The last type of episodic behavior pertinent to this discussion is
aggression in people with temporal lobe epilepsy. Patients with complex-partial seizures are more inclined to aggressive behavior (Bear,
1977) than are other neurologically impaired patients. Violence occurs
in a characteristic manner as a consequence of the powerful emotional
states which many of these patients experience. Aggression is not
necessarily explosive and is not triggered by trivial events in the manner
described above for patients with frontal lobe injury. It is not uncommon
for such a patient to remain angry for days. If the patient is violent, he
will not usually claim amnesia. While typically remorseful, he can still

detail the reasons for the anger. This pattern of lasting, self-justified, intense emotion leading to directed violence is the most common type of aggression in patients with complex-partial seizures in our experience. This is not the episodic dyscontrol syndrome (Mark and Ervin, 1970; Maletzky, 1973), a disorder of uncertain relationship to recognized brain disease. There are good experimental parallels in animals as well as depth electrode recording data in man (Mark and Ervin, 1970) which suggest that irritative lesions in the amygdala may be the basis for this episodic dyscontrol, but it is not clearly related to the clinical disorder of epilepsy (Bear, 1979).

CONCLUSIONS

Paroxysmal behavioral disorders may occur in many settings. This chapter has focused on several which are not epileptic but which might be or have been confused with epilepsy. For each disorder, a scheme for evaluation and treatment was suggested. As far as the evidence allowed, the mechanisms of these nonepileptic paroxysmal events were defined. Not all episodes of altered consciousness, transient amnesia, brief confusion, unusual movements or explosive outbursts are complex-partial seizures. Attention to the specific nature of the paroxysmal disorders should guide one to a correct diagnosis and management.

References

Transient Global Amnesia

Bender, M. B. Syndrome of isolated episode of confusion with amnesia. *J. Hillside Hosp.* 5:212–215, 1956.

Benson, D. F., Marsden, D., and Meadows, J. C. The amnesic syndrome of posterior cerebral artery occlusion. *Acta. Neurol. Scand.* 50:133–145, 1974.

Boudin, G., Pepin, B., Mikol, J., et al. Gliome du systeme limbique posterieur, revele par une amnesie globae transitoire: Observation anatomoclinique d'un cas. *Rev. Neurol.* 131:157–163, 1975.

DeJong, R. N., Itabashi, H. H. and Olson, J. R. Memory loss due to hippocampal lesions. *Arch. Neurol.* 20:339–348, 1969.

Evans, J. H. Transient loss of memory: An organic mental syndrome. *Brain* 89:539–548, 1966.

Fisher, C. M., and Adams, R. D. Transient global amnesia. *Acta. Neurol. Scand.* 40 (*suppl* 9):7–83, 1964.

Geschwind, N., and Fusillo, M. Color naming defects in association with alexia. *Arch. Neurol.* 15:137–146, 1966.

Gilbert, J. J., and Benson, D. F. Transient global amnesia: Report of two cases with definite etiologies. *J. Nerv. Ment. Dis.* 159:461–464, 1972.

Gordon, B. and Marin, O. S. M. Transient global amnesia: An extensive case report. *J. Neurol. Neurosurg. Psychiatry* 42:572–575, 1979.

Greene, H. H., and Bennett, D. R. Transient global amnesia with a previously unreported EEG abnormality. *Electroencephalogr. Clin. Neurophysiol.* 36:409–413, 1974.

Greenlee, J. E., Crampton, R. S., and Miller, J. Q. Transient global amnesia associated with cardiac arrhythmia and digitalis intoxication. *Stroke* 6:513–516, 1975.

Hartley, T. C., Heilman, K., and Garcia-Bengochia, F. A case of a transient global amnesia due to a pituitary tumor. *Neurology 24:*998–1000, 1974.

Heathfield, K. W. G., Croft, P. B., and Swash, M. The syndrome of transient global amnesia. *Brain 96:*729–736, 1973.

Lisak, R. P., and Zimmerman, R. A. Transient global amnesia due to a dominant hemisphere tumor. *Arch. neurol. 34:*317–318, 1975.

Lou, H. O. C. Repeated episodes of transient global amnesia. *Acta. Neurol. Scand. 44:*612–618, 1968.

Mathew, N. T., and Meyer, J. S. Pathogenesis and natural history of transient global amnesia. *Stroke 5:*303–311, 1974.

Mazzucchi, A., Moretti, G., Caffara, P., and Parma, M. Neuropsychological functions in the follow-up of transient global amnesia. *Brain 103:*161–178, 1980.

Milner, B., Corkin, S., and Teuber, H. H. Further analysis of the hippocampal amnestic syndrome: 14 year follow-up study of HM. *Neurophsychologia 6:*215–234, 1968.

Mumenthaler, M., Kaeser, H. E., Meyer, A., and Hess, T. Transient global amnesia after clioquinol. *J. Neurol. Neurosurg. Psychiatry 42:*1084–1090, 1979.

Nausieda, P. A., and Sherman, I. V. Long-term prognosis in transient global amnesia. *J.A.M.A. 241:*392–393, 1979.

Ponsford, J. L., and Donnan, G. A. Transient global amnesia: A hippocampal phenomenon? *J. Neurol. Neurosurg. Psychiatry 43:*285–287, 1980.

Poser, C. M., and Ziegler, D. Temporary amnesia as a manifestation of cerebrovascular insufficiency. *Trans. Am. Neurol. Assoc. 85:*221–223, 1960.

Rowan, J., and Protass, L. M. Transient global amnesia: Clinical and electroencephalographic findings in 10 cases. *Neurology 29:*869–872, 1979.

Shuping, J. R., Rollinson, R. D., and Toole, J. F. Transient global amnesia. *Ann. Neurol. 7:* 281–285, 1980.

Shuping, J. R., Toole, J. F., and Alexander, E., Jr. Transient global amnesia due to a glioma in the dominant hemisphere. *Neurology 30:*88–90, 1980.

Shuttleworth, E. C., and Wise, G. R. Transient global amnesia due to arterial embolism. *Arch. Neurol. 29:*340–342, 1973.

Steinmetz, E. F., and Vroom, F. Q. Transient global amnesia. *Neurology 22:*1193–1200, 1972.

Tharp, B. R. The electroencephalogram in transient global amnesia. *Electroencephalogr. Clin. Neurophysiol. 26:*96–99, 1969.

Victor, M., Adams, R. D., and Collins, G. H. *The Wernicke-Korsakoff Syndrome.* F. A. Davis Co., Philadelphia, 1971.

Victor, M., Angevine, J. B., Mancall, E. G., and Fisher, C. M. Memory loss with lesions of the hippocampal formation. *Arch. Neurol. 5:*244–263, 1961.

White, J. C., Langston, W., and Pedley, T. A. Benign epileptiform transients of sleep: Clarification of the small sharp spike controversy. *Neurology 27:*1061–1068, 1977.

Narcolepsy

Guilleminault, C., Brilliard, M., Montpalisir, J., and Dement, W. C. Altered states of consciousness in disorders of daytime sleepiness. *J. Neurol. Sci. 26:*377–393, 1975(a).

Guilleminault, C., Phillips, R., and Dement, W. C. A syndrome of hypersomnia with automatic behavior. *Electroencephalogr. Clin. Neurophysiol. 38:*403–413, 1975(b).

Parkes, J. D. A. The sleepy patient. *Lancet ii:*990–993, 1977.

Alcoholic Blackouts

Goodwin, D. W., Crane, J. B., and Guze, S. B. Alcoholic blackouts: A review and clinical study of 100 alcoholics. *Am. J. Psychiatry 126:*191–198, 1969(a).

Goodwin, D. W., Crane, J. B. and Guze, S. B. Phenomenological aspects of the alcoholic "blackout." *Br. J. Psychiatry 115:*1033–1038, 1969(b).

Tamerin, J. S., Weiner, S., Popper, R., et al. Alcohol and memory: Amnesia and short-term memory function during experimentally induced intoxication. *Am. J. Psychiatry 127:* 1659–1664, 1971.

Poriomania

Gastaut, H., Rober, J., and Roger, A. Sur la signification de certaines fugues épileptiques: A propos d'une observation électroclinique d'état de mal temporal. *Rev. Neurol.* 94:298–301, 1956.

Haller, W. F. Das Problem der Poriomania. *Nervenarzt* 9:385–389, 1957.

Kraeplin, E. *Psychiatrie.* Verlag Von Johann Ambrosius Barth, Leipzig, 1909.

Mayeux, R., Alexander, M. P., Benson, D. F., et al. Poriomania. *Neurology* 29:1616–1619, 1979.

Mayeux, R., and Lender, H. Complex partial status epilepticus: Case report and proposal for diagnostic criteria. *Neurology* 28:957–961, 1978.

Stengel, E. On the aetiology of fugue states. *J. Ment. Sci.* 87:572–599, 1941.

Stengel, E. Further studies on pathological wandering (fugue with the impulse to wander). *J. Ment. Sci.* 89:224–241, 1943.

Wells, C. E. Transient ictal psychosis. *Arch. Gen. Psychiatry* 32:1201–1203, 1975.

Migraine

Bickerstaff, E. R. Basilar artery migraine. *Lancet* i:15–17, 1961a.

Bickerstaff, E. R. Impairment of consciousness in migraine. *Lancet* ii:1057–1069, 1961b.

Bille, B. S. Migraine in school children. *Acta. Paediatr. Scand.* (*Suppl.*) 51:136, 1962.

Camfield, P. R., Metrakos, K., and Andermann, F. Basilar migraine, seizures and severe epileptiform EEG abnormalities. *Neurology* 28:584–588, 1978.

Connor, R. C. R. Complicated migraine. *Lancet* ii:1072–1075, 1962.

Ehyai, A. and Fenichel, G. M. The natural history of acute confusional migraine. *Arch. Neurol.* 35:368–369, 1978.

Emery, E. S. Acute confusional state in children with migraine. *Pediatrics* 60:110–114, 1977.

Gascon, G., and Barlow, C. Juvenile migraine, presenting as an acute confusional state. *Pediatrics* 45:628–635, 1970.

Golden, G. S., and French, J. H. Basilar artery migraine in young children. *Pediatrics* 56:722–726, 1975.

Hockaday, J. M., and Whitty, C. W. M. Factors determining the electroencephalogram in migraine: A study of 560 patients according to the clinical types of migraine. *Brain* 92:769–788, 1969.

Horenstein, S., Chamberlain, W., and Conomy, J. Infarction of the fusiform of the hippocampal formation and fusiform and lingual gyri. *Neurology* 24:1181–1183, 1974.

Lance, J. W., and Anthony, M. Some clinical aspects of migraine. *Arch. Neurol.* 15:356–361, 1966.

Lapkin, M. L., French, J. H., Golden, G. S., and Rowan, A. J. The electroencephalogram in childhood basilar artery migraine. *Neurology* 27:580–583, 1977.

Lees, F., and Watkins, S. M. Loss of consciousness in migraine. *Lancet* ii:647–650, 1963.

Medina, J. L., Rubino, F. A., and Ross, E. Agitated delirium caused by infarctions of the hippocampal formation and fusiform and lingual gyri. *Neurology* 24:1181–1183, 1974.

Mesulam, M. M., Waxman, S. G., and Geschwind, N., et al. Acute confusional state with right middle cerebral artery infarction. *J. Neurol. Neurosurg. Psychiatry* 39:84–89, 1976.

Pearce, J. M. S., and Foster, J. B. An investigation of complicated migraine. *Neurology* 15:333–340, 1965.

Riley, T. L., and Massey, E. W. The syndrome of aphasia, headaches and left temporal spikes. *Headache* 20:90–92, 1980.

Slatter, K. H. Some clinical and EEG findings in patients with migraine. *Brain* 91:85–98, 1968.

Swanson, J. W., and Vick, N. A. Basilar artery migraine. *Neurology* 28:782–786, 1978.

Acute Intermittent Porphyria

Becker, D. M., and Kramer, S. The neurological manifestations of porphyria: A review. *Medicine* 56:411–423, 1977.

Biagini, R., Tignani, A., Fifi, A. R., and Nappini, L. Acute intermittent porphyria and epilepsy. *Arch. Dis. Child.* 8:644–645, 1979.

Goldberg, A. Acute intermittent porphyria: A study of 50 cases. *Q. J. Med.* 110:183–209, 1959.

Sergay, S. M. Management of neurologic exacerbations of hepatic porphyria. *Med. Clin. North Am.* 63:453–463, 1979.

Stein, J. A., and Tschudy, D. P. Acute intermittent porphyria: A clinical and biochemical study of 46 patients. *Medicine* 49:1–16, 1970.

Tschudy, D. P., Valsamis, M., and Magnussen, C. R. Acute intermittent porphyria: Clinical and selected research aspects. *Ann. Intern. Med.* 83:851–864, 1975.

Waldenstrom, J. The porphyrias as inborn errors in metabolism. *Am. J. Med.* 22:758–773, 1957.

Paroxysmal Choreoathetosis

Arden, F. Idiopathic hypoparathyroidism. *Med. J. Aust.* 2:217–219, 1953.

Coulter, D. L., and Donofrio, P. Haloperidol for nonkinesiogenic paroxysmal dyskinesia. *Arch. Neurol.* 37:325–326, 1980.

Falconer, M. A., Driver, M. V., and Serafetinides, E. A. Seizures induced by movement: Report of a case relieved by operation. *J. Neurol. Neurosurg. Psychiatry* 26:300–307, 1963.

Goodenough, D. J., Fariello, R. G., Annis, B. L., and Chun, R. W. M. Familial and acquired paroxysmal dyskinesias. *Arch. Neurol.* 35:827–831, 1978.

Gowers, W. R. *Epilepsy and Other Chronic Convulsive Diseases: Their Causes, Symptoms, and Treatment*, ed. 2. London, J & A Churchill, Ltd., 1901, pp. 109–110.

Kato, M., and Araki, S. Paroxysmal kinesigenic choreoathetosis. *Arch. Neurol.* 20:508–513, 1969.

Kertesz, A. Paroxysmal kinesigenic choreoathetosis. *Neurology* 17:680–690, 1967.

Loong, S. C., and Ong, Y. Y. Paroxysmal kinesigenic choreoathetosis: A report of a case relieved by L-dopa. *J. Neurol. Neurosurg. Psychiatry* 36:921–924, 1973.

Mount, L. A., and Reback, S. Familial paroxysmal choreoathetosis: Preliminary report on a hitherto undescribed clinical syndrome. *Arch. Neurol. Psychiatry* 44:841–847, 1940.

Stevens, H. Paroxysmal choreoathetosis: A form of reflex epilepsy. *Arch. Neurol.* 14:415–420, 1966.

Suber, D., and Riley, T. L. Normal CT scan and valproic acid for paroxysmal kinesigenic choreoathetosis. *Arch. Neurol.* 37:327, 1980.

Tabaee-Zadeh, M. J., Frame, B., and Kapphahn, K. Kinesigenic choreoathetosis and idiopathic hypoparathyroidism. *N. Engl. J. Med.* 286:762–763, 1972.

Whitty, C. W. M., Lishman, W. A., and Fitzgibbon, J. P. Seizures induced by movement: A form of reflex epilepsy. *Lancet* 1:1403–1405, 1964.

Multiple Sclerosis

Andermann, F., Cosgrove, J. B. R., Lloyd-Smith, D., and Walter, A. M. Paroxysmal dysarthria and ataxia in multiple sclerosis. *Neurology* 9:211–215, 1959.

Ekborn, K. A., Westerberg, C. E., and Osterman, P. O. Focal sensory-motor seizures of spinal origin. *Lancet* i:67, 1968.

Espir, M. L. E., and Millac, P. Treatment of paroxysmal disorders in multiple sclerosis with carbamazepine. *J. Neurol. Neurosurg. Psychiatry* 33:528–531, 1970.

Espir, M. L. E., Watkins, S. M., and Smith, H. V. Paroxysmal dysarthria and other transient neurological disturbances in multiple sclerosis. *J. Neurol. Neurosurg. Psychiatry* 29:323–330, 1966.

Joynt, R. J., and Green, D. Tonic seizures as a manifestation of multiple sclerosis. *Arch. Neurol.* 6:292–299, 1962.

Matthews, W. B. Tonic seizures in disseminated sclerosis. *Brain* 81:193–206, 1958.

Matthews, W. B. Paroxysmal symptoms in multiple sclerosis. *J. Neurol. Neurosurg. Psychiatry* 38:617–623, 1975.

Miley, C. E., and Forster, F. M. Paroxysmal signs and symptoms in multiple sclerosis. *Neurology 24*:458–461, 1974.

Osterman, P. O., and Westerberg, C. E. Paroxysmal attacks in multiple sclerosis. *Brain 98*: 189–202, 1975.

Rasminsky, M. Ectopic generation of impulses and cross-talk in spinal nerve roots of "dystrophic" mice. *Ann. Neurol. 3*:351–357, 1978.

Seltzer, Z., and Devor, M. Ephaptic transmission in chronically damaged peripheral nerves. *Neurology 29*:1061–1064, 1979.

Fixed Neurological Disease

Bear, D. M. Temporal lobe epilepsy: A syndrome of sensory-limbic hyperconnection. *Cortex 15*:357–384, 1979.

Bear, D., and Fedio, P. Quantitative analysis of interictal behavior in temporal lobe epilepsy. *Arch. Neurol. 34*:454–467, 1977.

Damasio, A. The frontal lobes. In *Clinical Neuropsychology*, edited by Heilman, K. M., and Valenstein, E. Oxford University Press, New York, 1979.

Maletzky, B. M. The episodic dyscontrol syndrome. *Dis. Nerv. Syst. 34*:178–185, 1973.

Mark, V. K., and Ervin, F. R. *Violence and the Brain*. Harper & Row, New York, 1970.

EEG, INTENSIVE MONITORING, AND VIDEOTAPE

 # The Use of EEG in Pseudoseizures

DONALD F. SCOTT, F.R.C.P., D.P.M.

The use of the electroencephalograph (EEG) in the investigation of those suffering from epilepsy or suspected of having seizures remains controversial. Opinions vary from those who believe it to be of no value to those who use the EEG indiscriminately. A balanced view is obviously correct—employ this recording technique in an appropriate context, since the basic diagnosis of epilepsy must rest on the clinical aspects. It follows that the place of EEG methods in those suspected of having pseudoseizures is uncertain, but it is also a subject that has received little attention in its own right.

As we live in an age of high technology medicine, there is perhaps more difficulty in appreciating the use of the "straight forward" EEG for the diagnosis. Just as in the past when computer analysis techniques became available the possibilities of current methods had to be remembered, so now when telemetry (Binnie et al., 1981) and ambulatory monitoring techniques (Stores, 1980) as well as the simpler cerebral function monitoring apparatus (Prior, 1979) are readily available, it is necessary to bear in mind that visual inspection of the conventional paper trace still has value (Moffett and Scott, 1981). Such an idea was personally confirmed a few years ago when a female patient was referred with a diagnosis of hysterical deafness. A small dose of oral barbiturate produced light sleep, and repeated auditory stimuli failed to alter the recording. Subsequently it was shown that she had an unusual and severe form of progressive bilateral deafness. The usefulness of the straightforward EEG was further reinforced when another woman patient was referred with a diagnosis of pseudoseizures. On the first occasion she was obviously having a fit, and by inspection of the EEG the occurrence of a seizure discharge was clearly seen. About 2 years later she was referred again. Then, both by observation of the patient and by inspection of the EEG it was ascertained that this was not a fit.

There were no discharges in the recording and she recovered quickly, in contrast to the earlier occasion when there was confusion and postictal sleep.

In this chapter I shall attempt to evaluate the routine EEG in pseudoseizures, bearing in mind that other parameters like the electrocardiogram can be assessed simultaneously on the same paper trace. Further the EEG in patients with epilepsy is generally abnormal not only during but also between attacks, often a confirming factor when genuine seizures and pseudoseizures coexist. The possible role of triggering factors will also be considered, as well as the more sophisticated monitoring techniques.

THE ECG

It should not be forgotten that the ordinary EEG apparatus is quite capable of recording other physiological variables than brain potentials themselves. These can be helpful in determining whether an attack is in fact a seizure. Gastaut and Broughton (1972) have shown that there is an alteration both in heart rate and in respiration when a seizure occurs.

The most common change is tachycardia; sometimes bradycardia is noted, and very occasionally cardiac standstill occurs. The former is the only likely change that could accompany pseudoseizures. Hence when there is doubt about the nature of the attack the technician should always be instructed to monitor the cardiograph simultaneously with the EEG at least for part of the test. Clearly a full ECG is inappropriate but in our experience a classical Lead I is easy to apply and can yield useful information. A number of reports, see for example Selby and Driver (1977), have indicated unusual changes in the cardiograph which have been diagnostic. If there is real doubt about the rhythmical integrity of the heart the ECG can be monitored for 24 hours in the same way as the EEG using a cassette recorder, a technique mentioned later.

SOME LIMITATIONS OF THE EEG

It is quite clear that there are various constraints associated with the recording of electrical brain activity. Limitations are present in terms of spatial and temporal sampling. It represents a narrow-angle snapshot of the CNS, and seizure discharges may not be observed on the scalp but can be seen clearly in depth recordings (Chatrian and Chapman, 1960), a problem that must be considered in the EEG of pseudoseizure patients. Emphasis must always be placed on the actual observation of an attack (Rodin et al., 1955) or as accurate an eyewitness account as is possible (see Chapter 2).

Another aspect is the abnormality that may be seen in the interseizure

EEG in patients with a psychiatric disorder who may or may not be suffering from seizures. Personality disorder and schizophrenia are two such conditions (Schwartz and Scott, 1975). This abnormality may also occur unexpectedly in other conditions, for example, in anorexia nervosa.

DISCHARGES DURING AND BETWEEN GENUINE SEIZURES

To interpret the EEG with certainty in pseudoseizure patients, it is important to make a clear-cut distinction between those features seen in the recording *during* seizures and those which occur *between* seizures. The true seizure is usually characterized by repetitive spikes, occurring either focally and then becoming generalized (depending on the underlying pathology) or commencing in a generalized fashion. However, there are marked differences in wave form and frequency seen. Thus, an apparent alpha frequency activity observed in one location and spreading widely may well indicate that a fit is beginning there and spreading. The term "subclinical seizure discharges" is a helpful shorthand in those instances in which there are no clear-cut clinical manifestations and in which alterations presumably would be found if simultaneous behavioral testing was possible. A problem arises in a few instances in which definite seizures are witnessed by the clinician but there are no electroencephalographic concomitants. These are rare, although depth recordings (Chatrian and Chapman, 1960) support the view that this does occur. It is however most unusual in our experience for the EEG to remain totally normal during an actual seizure. At the very least, alpha activity is attenuated, beta components are reduced, and postictal localized or generalized slow activity is seen.

Of more importance in ordinary EEG work is the fact that there are clear-cut signs of epilepsy *between* seizures. Thus spikes, sharp waves or complexes occur in a localized or generalized fashion and confirm the clinical diagnosis in many cases. However, these features may be seen in other conditions, for example, after head injury or subarachnoid hemorrhage in the absence of a seizure. Nevertheless the observations of Zivin and Marsan (1968), that seizures may subsequently occur in neurological patients with this type of EEG abnormality, must be heeded.

WHAT CHANGES OCCUR DURING PSEUDOSEIZURES?

There are two main aspects to be taken into account (Table 6.1). Firstly, the actual brain activity recorded and, secondly, the muscle and other artifacts observed in the tracing. The first is obviously quite

Table 6.1
Main EEG Aspects to be Considered

1. Are there definite abnormalities between attacks?
   Spikes, sharp waves or complexes
2. What happens when an attack occurs?
   Seizure discharge, type of artifact
3. Type of postattack changes?
   Alpha rhythm returns quickly, slow activity, localized reduction of fast elements

different in the pseudoseizure than in a genuine fit. No spikes or other rhythmical seizure elements are seen; sometimes although rarely, inter-seizure forms such as localized sharp waves and complexes may continue during the attack, but these are often difficult to discern because of artifact. Alpha activity may continue even in a rhythmical form throughout the whole of the pseudoseizure but it is usually impossible to discern because of the masking effect of artifact. In any case the patient may open his/her eyes, thus blocking the alpha activity. The recording of the attack itself will therefore often be featureless.

The duration should be considered. This of itself may not be very helpful because of the variable length of seizures, particularly those of temporal lobe type which often give rise to the greatest difficulties in the separation of genuine seizures from pseudoseizures. A useful point is the timing of EEG changes and the behavioral events. They may not correspond; for example, disturbance of speech may be discrepant compared with alterations in the EEG (Bickford, 1979).

Secondly, considering artifact, that seen in a fit tends to be organized in clusters of muscle spikes in relation to the underlying convulsive seizure discharge. In a pseudoseizure the picture is clouded by the gross and varying movement disturbance. Even if clusters of muscle activity appear, they are seen randomly: now on one side of the head, then on the other, now anteriorly, then posteriorly—difficult to understand in neurophysiological terms. This corresponds to the clinical observation that movements may affect at one moment the right arm, then suddenly the left leg. The way the artifact disappears is also important—not a gradually slowing and decreasing intensity as the underlying brain discharges subside, but rather there is often a sudden end.

Perhaps most important is the postattack period. Here, in the pseudoseizure patient alpha activity returns immediately and in abundance if the eyes remain shut. Such a feature is extremely rare following a true seizure even of a brief complex partial-temporal lobe type. In addition in these cases, although the record can be of low voltage, slow activity is seen, sometimes localized or more widespread. Careful examination of fast components can also be helpful. Is there localized reduction in an area where the attack appeared to commence? Such a change would not be observed after a pseudoseizure. A confusing feature may be found in those patients with definite epilepsy, complicated by pseudoseizures. The interictal phenomena such as spikes, sharp waves and complexes may reappear within a few seconds or, more commonly, within a few minutes after the attack subsides. However, this must be weighed in combination with all the other elements on the EEG tracing to establish a definite diagnosis.

OTHER EEG OBSERVATIONS

Routine activation procedures possibly with additional electrodes must be considered (Table 6.2), nevertheless the technician's observations during the test are of great importance. He/she should always be instructed to note the attitude of the patient; also, apart from the patient's state of consciousness, any obvious clinical abnormalities and details of attacks that occur should be noted. This can be particularly useful when there is any question, for example, of hyperventilation attacks. The technician then is warned not only to observe the patient carefully but also to make sure the tracing is as satisfactory as possible.

Hyperventilation is routinely performed except in those patients who may have raised intracranial pressure or other conditions in which untoward effects may occur with this procedure, which provokes relative cerebral hypoxia. This technique may cause a definite attack of petit mal or temporal lobe type and confirm that the condition is epilepsy. As hyperventilation leads to respiratory alkalosis, tetany with the usual posturing of the hands may result, particularly if the procedure is well done. Should this be the case and there is no alteration in the appearance of spike and wave in the EEG, then petit mal can confidently

Table 6.2
EEG Provocative Techniques

1. What happens with overbreathing?
   Spike and wave, attack provoked
2. Does photic stimulation produce a change?
   An attack, spike and wave, artifact only
3. Is a sleep recording justified?
   Normal electrical phenomena, seizure discharge, abreaction
4. Should nasopharyngeal or sphenoidal electrodes be used?
   Temporal lobe or other localized discharges

be excluded. The normal changes evoked, namely episodic delta activity, in young individuals subside rapidly, but any focal or generalized "epileptic activity" may persist for minutes. Sometimes overbreathing provokes an attack which the patient says subsequently is one of her usual spells, thus confirming the diagnosis of a pseudoseizure.

Photic stimulation is almost invariably performed as part of the routine EEG. Responses appear symmetrically over the posterior head regions, generally of 30–100 μv. However, in patients with attacks produced by viewing television or exposed to flashing lights in the environment, the evoked components are of very high voltage, generalized and of spike and wave type, and persisting after the flash stimulus is discontinued. This is seen in true cases of photically induced reflex epilepsy. Should such a response occur, then it is quite obvious that the patient has genuine seizures, although of course pseudoseizures triggered in various ways may also occur in the same patient.

Assuming that nothing untoward emerges with these routine activations, consideration should then be given to the use of oral hypnotic drugs to produce sleep during the EEG (Scott, 1975). These should always be employed when the clinician feels that the diagnosis is that of epilepsy, rather than of any other disorder. Sleep tracings may provoke temporal lobe or other focal changes. In patients with pseudoseizures, only normal sleep phenomena are seen but abreaction by the drugs given may occur. Many centers still use barbiturate compounds, although benzodiazepines are employed by others. Intravenous barbiturates such as methohexitone or Pentothal are quicker in producing sleep and EEG changes. Another procedure is sleep deprivation. The patient, child or adult, has to be awake for the night prior to the recording, and the resulting activation of discharges in the EEG can be very rewarding.

If all these procedures still fail to produce positive evidence for or against the diagnosis of pseudoseizures, then the question of nasopharyngeal or sphenoidal electrodes has to be considered. In our experience however, if all other EEGs are normal or show very minor features then these techniques are unlikely to be rewarding. In particular, yield of positive results in patients with normal sleep recordings is minimal (Prior et al., 1976).

TRIGGER FACTORS

A proportion of patients report that there are specific triggers to attacks. These include those in whom the spells appear to be pseudoseizures as well as others in whom it seems likely that the epilepsy is of genuine type—true reflex epilepsy. A careful history is valuable here.

Patients who have definite seizures usually give a fairly specific account of the precipitation; for example, they occur with watching television or more rarely with complex patterned stimuli, reading material or music (Scott, 1977). In these instances, replication of the appropriate stimulus can be provocative in the EEG laboratory. This is not always true, even when the tracing is abnormal between attacks and strongly suggests that their account is of a genuine nature. Presumably, the unusual situation with observers and tethering to apparatus mitigates against producing an attack.

The pseudoseizure patient often describes unusual and rather variable provocative stimuli which can rarely be reproduced in the laboratory and which virtually never elicit seizure discharge or a fit. Patients who say that traffic noise, typing or electric razors will all produce attacks usually do not display this under test conditions even if they say that the stimuli as presented are of appropriate type. As Liske and Forster (1964) pointed out, unusual stimuli in unusual situations are generally suspect. Another approach is to use intravenous convulsants to bring on an attack. These almost invariably fail, but in any case the record produced is so artifact ridden that interpretation is almost impossible.

MONITORING SYSTEMS

If the conventional techniques so far described do not produce positive results, it has to be clearly decided whether the evidence is strongly suggestive of genuine seizures or pseudoseizures. Should the former seem likely then various monitoring systems are available to help resolve the problem (Table 6.3). The simplest and cheapest is the cerebral function monitor (Prior, 1979). A single channel compressed and processed recording can show when a fit occurs; a sudden short upswing of activity is clearly seen even by the uninitiated. Such a method can help in the separation of true seizures from pseudoseizures. However, the patient has to be attached with wires to the apparatus so the more sophisticated procedures, even though more expensive, have

Table 6.3
Monitoring Procedures

1. Cerebral function monitor?
    Patient attached with leads, easy interpretation, relatively cheap
2. Telemetry with or without video?
    Prolonged, in hospital, expensive
3. Ambulatory monitoring?
    24 hours or more, quick review, home or hospital

advantages. Telemetry, in which the patient's EEG is broadcast to the pick-up apparatus, seems a practical alternative. The brain recording can be displayed on the split-screen television monitor, the other half being a video recording of the patient showing the simultaneous behavioral state (Sato et al., 1976). This is valuable in difficult cases but, apart from the cost, the system collects large amounts of data which can be time-consuming to analyze. It also has a limited range and therefore requires hospital admission away from the patient's home environment. Hence the advantage of the ambulatory monitoring system now used widely (Stores, 1980). A cassette is able to record not only EEG but also various physiological parameters, and hours or days of variables can be stored on such a tape and scanned rapidly.

The record obtained is of high quality and can be assessed in an uncomplicated manner, without access to computer facilities. Head-mounted preamplifiers attached to the electrodes allow the reduction of movement artifact, and the battery cassette is easily concealed on the patient's clothing. One of the four available channels marks clinical events and when the playback is viewed this can be used as an auditory signal to indicate the part of the EEG to be examined in detail. Thus seizure discharges, their appearance, and spread are rapidly assessed. The method is obviously of great value in those patients in whom pseudoseizures are suspected, and in those patients in whom there is a possibility of cerebral attacks triggered by a heart arrhythmia the ECG can be monitored in addition.

CONCLUSION

As always the diagnosis of pseudoseizures rests heavily on clinical information. However, the conventional EEG may afford valuable support, for or against the physicians' views. The tracing before, during and after a presumed seizure must be studied carefully. If there still remains doubt about the diagnosis, monitoring for longer periods than is possible with conventional EEG should be carefully considered. It must be affirmed that even after these procedures have been carried out there often remains in some patients doubt about the true diagnosis.

References

Bickford, R.G. Activation procedures and special electrodes. In *Current Practice of Clinical Electroencephalography*, edited by Klass, D.W., and Darby, D.D. Raven Press, New York, 1979.
Binnie, C.D., Rowan, A.J., Overweg, J., Meinardi, H., Wisonsin, J., Kamp, A., and Lopez du Silva, F. A clinical evaluation of tetermetric EEG and video monitoring in epilepsy. *Neurology*, 1981, in press.
Chatrian G.E., and Chapman, W.P. Electrographic study of the amygdaloid region with implanted electrodes in patients with temporal lobe epilepsy. In *Electrical Studies of*

the Anaesthetised Brain, edited by Ramey, E.R. and O'Doherty, D.S. Hoeber Medical, Harper, New York, 1960.

Gastaut, H., and Broughton, R. *Epileptic Seizures: Clinical and Electrographic Features, Diagnosis and Treatment*. Charles C Thomas, Springfield, IL, 1972.

Liske, E., and Forster, F.M. Pseudoseizures: A problem in diagnosis and management of epileptic patients. *Neurology 41*:41–49, 1964.

Moffett, A., and Scott, D.F. The EEG in the diagnosis of hysterical attacks in patients with epilepsy. *Electroencephalogr. Clin. Neurophysiol. 51*:52, 1981.

Prior, P.F., Maynard, D.E., and Scott, D.F. The value of sphenoidal recordings in patients with temporal lobe epilepsy. In *Proceedings of Seventh International Symposium on Epilepsy*, edited by Franz, D. Georg Thieme, Stuttgart, 1976.

Prior, P.F. *Monitoring Cerebral Function*. Elsevier North Holland, Amsterdam, 1979.

Rodin, E.A., Mulder, D.W., Faucett, R.L., and Bickford, R.G. Psychological factors in convulsive disorders of focal origin. *Arch. Neurol. Psychiatry 74*:365–374, 1955.

Sato, S., Penry, J.K., and Dreifuss, F.G. Electroencephalographic monitoring of generalised spike-and-wave paroxysms in the hospital ward and at home. In *Quantitative Analytical Studies in Epilepsy*, edited by Kelloway, P., and Petersen, I. Raven Press, New York, 1976.

Schwartz, M., and Scott, D.F. EEG features of depressive and schizophrenic states. *Br. J. Psychiatry 126*:408–413, 1975.

Scott, D.F. Musicogenic epilepsy. In *Music and the Brain*, edited by Critchley, MacD., and Henson, R.A. Heinemann, London, 1977.

Scott, D.F. *Understanding EEG*. Lippincott, Philadelphia, 1975.

Selby, P.J., and Driver, M.V. An unusual case of apparent epilepsy: ECG and EEG in a case of Jervell Lange-Neilson syndrome. *J. Neurol. Neurosurg. Psychiatry 40*:1102–1108, 1977.

Stores, G. Ambulatory EEG monitoring in the diagnosis of epilepsy. *J. Intern. Biomed. Inform. Data 1*:1–7, 1980.

Zivin, L., and Marsan, C. A. Incidence and prognostic significance of epileptiform activity in the EEG in non-epileptic subjects. *Brain 91*:751–778, 1968.

Chapter 7

Videotape Recording in Epilepsy and Pseudoseizures

ROBERT G. FELDMAN, M.D.
NORMAN L. PAUL, M.D.
JACKIE CUMMINS-DUCHARME, M.S.W.

Clinical manifestations of seizures or other alterations of consciousness often are experienced by the subject without observers. If not recalled, events may be totally unretrievable even by history. Semipurposeful activities or automatic behaviors, even when observed and described by witnesses, may be recalled or described with remarkable inaccuracies. The astonishment of watching a seizure easily leads to exaggerations or misinterpretation of the behaviors displayed by the patient. There is great value in having a correct and accurate description of the seizure, the nature of its onset, development and resolution, as well as the total duration of the episode and postictal state. When the diagnosis is in doubt, a careful characterization is helpful, but a permanent videotape recording (VTR) of the event provides even better documentation of the phenomenon, especially when the recorded behavior can be correlated with the electroencephalographic (EEG) data.

VIDEOTAPE DOCUMENTATION OF EPILEPTIC SEIZURES

Simultaneous EEG and videotape recording produces a clinical-physiological-time documentation of behavior (Ajmone-Marsan and Abraham, 1960; Bowden et al., 1975). Using special techniques provides a way to correlate EEG with behavior in the freely moving subject (Ives et al., 1973; Porter et al., 1971). The procedure focuses one camera on the patient, who is wired with electrodes connected either to a telemeter transmitter or by cable to an electroencephalograph; a second camera is focused on the EEG write-out. The picture of the patient and the simultaneous EEG tracing appear on a split-screen videomonitor. This combined recording is stored on the videotape for future analysis and interpretation.

Penry et al. (1975) established the value of this technique by discriminating a group of patients with generalized epilepsy of the absence type from those with complex partial epilepsy (CPE). Additional data came from a very complete analysis of psychomotor attacks and EEG correlates by Delgado-Escueta and his associates (1977), whose studies of lapse of consciousness and automatisms in complex partial epilepsy expanded the earlier work of Ajmone-Marsan and Abraham (1960). Delgado-Escueta et al. (1977) defined mainly two electroclinical types of psychomotor attacks. The first and most common type has three clinical phases: 1) motionless stare, 2) stereotyped movements and 3) reactive automatisms during impaired consciousness. In the first type, focal temporal or lateralizing phenomena are noted in the EEG. The second type of attack in CPE begins with a stereotyped reactive automatism, associated with diffuse changes in the EEG. In a later study of 406 attacks, Delgado-Escueta et al. (1979) concluded that videotaping analysis of complex partial epilepsy provided 1) a means for identifying states of an attack and its mode of presentation, 2) documentation and quantification of seizures and 3) a method for differentiating epileptic twilight states from other forms of mental confusion in fugue states. Using depth electrodes with this technique, focal depth discharges were found to precede the first manifestations of the clinical attack during complex partial seizures; in generalized epilepsy, clinical attacks might be recorded on videotape before the diffuse bifrontal EEG patterns are recorded. Clinical attacks of unconsciousness may appear simultaneously with or follow partial frontal or frontothalamic patterns. The information gathered by these studies enables clinicians to relate the clinical observations to probable electrocerebral events.

VIDEOTAPE AND EEG RECORDING IN DIFFERENTIATION OF EPILEPSY FROM PSEUDOSEIZURE

The physician who is faced with the question of "Is this a real seizure?" depends upon his judgement of what he sees or what is described to him. The classical description of hysterical seizures (elsewhere in this volume) has permitted the use of the features of the clinical "seizure" to make the diagnosis. Often, it is the inclination of the physician to "want" to make an organic diagnosis when a purely psychogenic one is more than justifiable and deserves primary therapy. In nonepileptic disorders or pseudoseizures, excessive antiepileptic medications not only are unnecessary but also further obscure the issues by clouding the sensorium of the patient. Early and correct diagnosis of the nonepileptic "seizures" is important. Videotape documentation with EEG correlation is a useful tool and provides important data in making a clinical analysis and in planning appropriate treatment.

It is possible that epileptic-like behavior occurs in patients whose surface EEGs are normal but whose depth EEGs are confirmatory of epilepsy. Likewise, nonepileptics with normal EEGs may exhibit episodic behaviors of psychological origins. Additionally, there are those who have combinations of both epileptic seizures and motivationally determined disturbances of behavior. The epilepsy-like physical expression perhaps develops in the epileptic patients because they have learned a pattern of behavior which "solves problems" for them. Differentiation of which type of seizure is actually occurring, real or simulated, requires careful analysis of the clinical phenomena. Videotape with or without EEG monitoring is very helpful.

It was concluded from a study of 9 epileptic patients who were suspected of having coexistent hysterical seizures that VTR-EEG monitoring is useful in differential diagnosis and, therefore, in treatment (Ramani et al., 1980). From the analysis of VTRs, these authors found that an hysterical seizure is not a homogeneous unitary disorder but is a complex symptom with diverse psychosocial determinants (conversion reaction is a more appropriate diagnostic term for these seizures). In addition to clarifying the diagnosis, the information gathered on the VTR was used in family therapy groups to help neutralize the problems and alleviate the need for "using" seizures as a mechanism for coping.

Detailed VTR-EEG recordings help differentiate between psychotic behaviors and epileptic phenomenon as well. Hallucinations, dissociative reactions, dysphoric states and paranoid ideation may occur in psychotic as well as epileptic persons with schizophreniform psychosis associated with some forms of epilepsy (Slater et al., 1964). Gladwell et al. (1979) described a 15-year-old girl who began to exhibit "uncooperative behavior" at age 2½. She was described as "manipulative" and "hysterical" throughout her preadolescence. She began to complain about seeing flashing lights and the image of a "little man digging into her eye"; she said that she was being chased by green monsters. When admitted to the hospital for psychiatric evaluation, she showed variable levels of consciousness; talk was coherent for short periods of time, but in "baby talk." In this case, conditions which were related to ictal activity were differentiated from those in which psychological symptoms were primary. Successful differentiation of epileptic twilight states from psychotic fugue states was also done by Belafsky et al. (1978). In their 3 case studies, VTR-EEG analysis showed that confusion, automatic behavior, amnesia, speech arrest and continuous epileptiform paroxysms were the cardinal features of epileptic twilight states.

We have used videotape techniques in subjects who had evidence that emotional stress may be a contributing factor in poor seizure control and to differentiate "real seizures" from pseudoseizures. The procedure includes several phases. In the initial phase of the study, there are interviews to confirm the neurologic background and case history of recurrent seizures; the age of onset, clinical manifestations, frequency of recurrence, duration and previous treatments are noted. During this exploratory phase, a thorough psychosocial assessment is completed to determine if there are environmental, interpersonal or intrapsychic stresses that could be associated with the "triggering" of seizure activity. Electroencephalographic recording is done for a 24-hour period, including the time of a videotaped interview. In this way a correlation can be made with possibly stressful material and seizure activity. The patient is videotaped while the EEG is recorded on a tape recorder ambulatory pack (Medilog-Oxford). If a "seizure" is experienced by the subject, he/she is instructed to push a button on the recording pack signalling a point in time on the EEG recording which can be correlated with the same time on the videopicture, thereby relating observed behavior seen on VTR with electrographic data on the ambulatory EEG monitor. Some patients are interviewed in the laboratory, and both the patient and the EEG are videotaped during the interview. In addition to the subjective reporting of the patient, observations are made by the physician and social worker present during the interview. Interpretation of the EEG and its correlation with the videotape recordings are done at a later time. The results of this technique in two subjects are described below.

During the interview session, the patient is asked to talk about his/her seizure, family, events and other topics which they believe contribute to their "seizures." Stressor topics (audio and video) are presented to the subject in an effort to provoke emotional responses and to stimulate recall of possibly emotionally upsetting thoughts or feelings. This confrontation technique has been described previously in our study of emotionally triggered epilepsy (Feldman and Paul, 1976). In the patients with a questionable diagnosis of epilepsy versus pseudoseizures, the videotape recording of "epileptiform behavior" and the results of the EEG are reviewed with the patient. The confrontation video playback is then used to show the patient what he/she looked like during a seizure. The nonepileptic nature of the movements or behavior is pointed out along with normal EEG data. The therapist attempts to relate the occurrence of the apparent emotionally determined basis for the seizure-like actions and behavior and seeks to provide insight and instruction to the patient and family about the use of more effective ways of dealing with emotional conflict.

The following case summaries illustrate the application of this procedure to clinical problems of differentiating epileptic phenomena from pseudoseizures.

Case 1

A 12-year-old male had a generalized convulsion with loss of consciousness. Although minor absence spells with myoclonic jerks of limbs occurred when he was sleep deprived or emotionally upset, he had no other large seizures for the next 10 years while receiving 400 mg of phenytoin and 750 mg of methsuximide daily. Since seizures were not a problem for him, he did not take medication regularly.

At age 29, the patient was referred for reevaluation because of an increasing number of "absence-type" spells, Moreover, he had become more withdrawn, experiencing periodic depression and anxiety attacks. The referral requested a determination of these episodic behaviors; namely, were they psychogenic or uncontrolled seizures. Several routine electroencephalograms were "normal" and the clinical impression was that his "seizures" were not epileptic in origin.

It was learned that before the onset of his seizures, he had been his mother's favorite. He reportedly had excelled in school and said he had an I.Q. "above 180." He described his father as both passive and unsuccessful and his mother as overprotective, the dominant force in the family. After his first seizure, he was no longer deemed the "perfect" child, and he reported that he was then devalued and criticized. He reported that he had no "real friends" and felt like an "unsuccessful" child.

During a videotape interview with a 24-hour EEG recording, a stressor audio tape was presented consisting of an exchange between a woman and her adult daughter who expressed anger at the mother for making her feel devalued and unappreciated. The daughter told the mother that unrealistic demands created burdens in the past which persisted in the present. The mother defended herself by stating her intention was to protect her daughter, and she expressed surprise at the daughter's feelings.

Although there were no clinical seizures observed during the interview session, analysis of the 24-hour EEG ambulatory monitor revealed definite abnormalities which appeared 10 minutes after the presentation of the stressor tape and during the patient's verbal attack upon his parents. There were paroxysmal bursts of high amplitude 3 Hz spikes and waves, but there was no observable seizure behavior.

Comment. This recorded interview of a stress-inducing conversation served as a means for documenting the relationship between this patient's "spells" and emotional factors. Without EEG monitoring, the burst of bioelectrical seizure activity would have been missed. A briefer EEG may have detected the spikes and would have been labelled "normal." The seizures required more drug therapy and were not mere psychological lapses. Additionally, family therapy with both parents was recommended and instituted, which neutralized some of the anxiety that led to seizures during stress. Methsuximide was increased to 1000 mg/day, with elimination of staring spells and jerking movements of limbs.

Case 2

An 18-year-old female developed spells diagnosed as partial complex seizures, consisting of staring, tightening of muscles and "losing touch" with others. Previous EEG recordings were normal and medications were ineffective in controlling her episodic behaviors. Additionally, she reported many emotional difficulties around "separations," beginning at age 8 when her mother deserted the family. The VTR-EEG recording was introduced to help make a differential diagnosis and to determine the "emotional" triggers. During the VTR-EEG recording, she attempted to walk out of the room, stating she could not tolerate seeing herself during the videotape replay; she said she looked like her mother. The patient reported that she had two seizures following the interview, one approximately 20 minutes following the actual session and another approximately 1 hour later. No one observed these spells and the 24-hour EEG, which had been monitoring her electro-cerebral activity during this time, recorded no seizure discharge.

Comment. The 24-hour EEG monitor and videotape interview helped to establish the diagnosis of pseudoseizure and rule out epilepsy in this subject. Her anticonvulsant medication was discontinued. The VTR of the interview was reviewed with her several times, with a concomitant discussion of her fears and feelings. As she was able to verbalize her fears of abandonment and loss, she began to recognize that in the past she "needed to have the seizures." Two months following the interview, L.S. wrote a letter of thanks and told how she was getting along without "seizures," in spite of various chaotic episodes in her life.

The VTR-EEG recording provided data comparing subjective and observable behaviors to electrocerebral events and reinforced the clinical impression that the patient was not having epileptic attacks but rather was having pseudoseizures.

To make an organic diagnosis without clear evidence of epilepsy has serious iatrogenic biopsychosocial ramifications for the patient in long-term effects of medications and the reinforced stigma of epilepsy. The VTR-EEG recording can be useful in delineating the pseudoseizure from epileptic phenomenon. If the patient has epileptic seizures, appropriate treatment can then be instituted. Whether the patient has pseudoseizures or epilepsy, the identification of relevant emotional triggers may aid the patient in coping with the threatening environmental cues.

USE OF VTR IN IDENTIFYING EMOTIONAL TRIGGERS OF EPILEPTIC SEIZURES

In some cases, postictal amnesia prevents a patient from remembering the circumstances and emotional triggers leading to a seizure. Various behavioral techniques may be useful in treating specific patients with seizure disorder (Feldman et al., 1982). Behavioral methods include the application of psychodynamic theory, learning theory and biofeedback theory. The behavioral paradigm of stimulus-organism-response (S-O-R) delineates three theoretical targets that are useful in understanding and treating seizures: 1) the seizure as a response to specific internal and external stimuli (S), 2) the seizure as a reinforced (R) behavior, and 3) the seizure as an underlying conflict within the individual (O) (Feldman and Ricks, 1978). Moreover, the VTR facilitates behavioral methods in decreasing the frequency of seizures and episodic behaviors.

When the seizure is a response to a specific environmental cue, the focus is on the precipitating event or trigger in the S-O-R model. Identification of the trigger is essential in altering the seizure threshold through manipulation of the stimulus. The specific behavioral techniques used to distinguish the cue as a trigger of seizures are 1) systematic desensitization, 2) habituation, 3) relaxation, 4) conditioning, 5) adversive conditioning and 6) biofeedback-sensorimotor rhythm training. Some patients who are able to identify the triggering stimulus experience better control using these techniques. Through stimulated recall and videotape or audio presentation of emotionally laden stressors, seizures were induced. Once able to identify and acknowledge the stressor, the subject learned to 1) avoid events that could elicit seizures and 2) cope with stressful environmental cues. The VTR facilitates this process by delineating the antecedent event which precipitates the seizure activity. Then, with use of VTR playback, feedback of the stimulus and the organism's response to it can be associated. The noxious stimulus then may be deconditioned or desensitized; the patient is provided with a conscious awareness which neutralizes the trigger.

In the S-O-R chain, the seizure may be a reinforced behavior. In this aspect, the consequences of seizures are emphasized. The frequency of some seizures depends upon the responses elicited by oversolicitous others following a seizure. Some patients learn that a seizure will elicit attention, and this can increase the frequency of seizures. Behavioral methods have been used to reduce the seizure frequency by changing the reinforcement. The VTR can help the patient's significant others observe their reactions as a contributing, reinforcing factor. Moreover, as the patient views his own seizure, the reinforced consequences may diminish.

The seizure may also be a symptom of an underlying conflict in the organism of the S-O-R paradigm. The recurrence of seizures diminishes self-confidence in a patient whose epilepsy is poorly controlled. He is dependent upon others during the attack when consciousness is affected. Frequently, the patient feels ashamed and is fearful of rejection by significant others. The patient believes he has no control over his environment or his responses to it. During stressful times, some patients with seizures have semipurposeful behaviors. The behaviors are seen as manipulative. These behavioral patterns often develop as a result of an accumulation of learned responses to environmental and interpersonal cues. In this model, psychodynamic techniques are used, focusing on the personality structure and defense mechanisms. Although there is an identification of emotional triggers, these cues reflect unresolved conflicts. Thus, the stimuli are seen thematically rather than as specific entities. Many patients have negative misconceptions of their physical state during their seizure activity (Feldman, 1982). The negative self-image has psychosocial ramifications which may create intrapsychic conflicts. The VTR playback narrows the discrepancy between his projected perceptions of the seizure event and the validated actuality of what has been recorded. For some patients, postictal amnesia prevents the patient from remembering the stimulus which induced the seizure activity. The VTR playback "reminds" the patient of the cues and concomitant themes. This assists the patient in understanding his underlying conflicts. As the patient gains greater control over these triggers and conflicts, the frequency of seizures may decrease (Fig. 7.1).

The videotape documentation with or without EEG correlates is a useful instrument to aid the patient and the patient's family. With the EEG, it can correlate subjective and observable behavior with electrocerebral events. Control of seizures is affected by the individual's behavior and attitude. The VTR pinpoints the areas of stress which may exacerbate the frequency of seizures or elicit motivationally determined episodic behavior. The VTR can help prepare patients to cope with the environmental stressors through stimulated recall and videotape replay. Finally, VTR in epileptology is very useful in providing documentation of the seizure and in capturing some of the emotional aspects of treatment for students and practitioners.

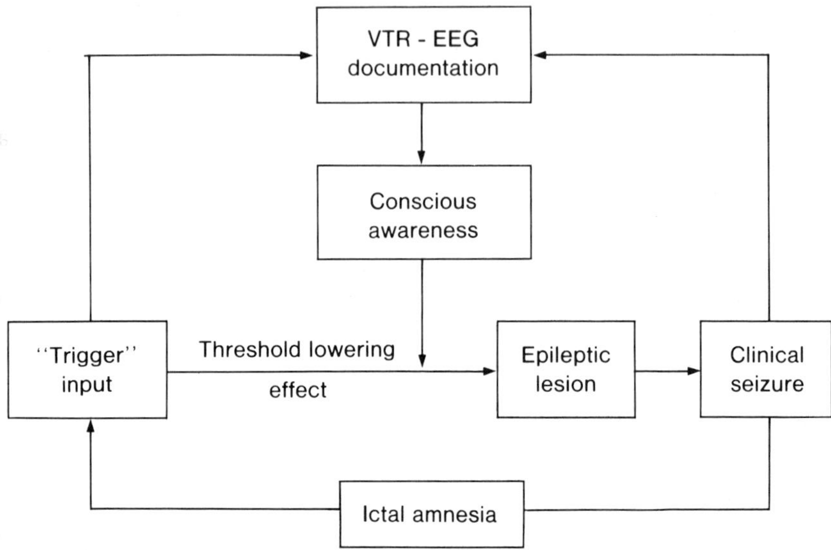

Figure 7.1.   A component model to describe the relationship of specific triggers or inputs of stimuli or emotional experiences which lower the threshold of a susceptible epileptic. The subsequent occurrence of a clinical attack and the ictal amnesia eliminate the antecedent events from recall. Videotape recording provides this information upon replay after an induced seizure. Once incorporated as conscious awareness of the relationship between the trigger and the seizure, the threshold lowering impact is lessened or even interrupted, often preventing some seizures.

References

Ajmone-Marsan, C., and Abraham, K. A seizure atlas. *Electroencephalogr. Clin. Neurophysiol. 15*(suppl.):215, 1960.

Belafsky, M.A., et al. Prolonged epileptic twilight states: Continuous recordings with nasopharyngeal electrodes and videotape analysis. *Neurology 28*:239, 1978.

Bowden, A.N., Fitch, P., and Willison, R.G. The place of EEG telemetry and closed-circuit television in the diagnosis and management of epileptic patients. *Proc. Roy. Soc. Med 68*:246, 1975.

Delgado-Escueta, A.V., Kunze, U., Waddell, G., et al. Lapse of consciousness and automatisms in temporal lobe epilepsy: A videotape analysis. *Neurology 27*:144, 1977.

Delgado-Escueta, A.V., Nashold, B., Freedman, M., et al. Videotaping epileptic attacks during stereoelectroencephalography. *Neurology 29*:473, 1979.

Feldman, R.G. Complex partial seizures. In *Epilepsy: Diagnosis and Management*, edited by Browne, T.R., and Feldman, R.G. Little, Brown, Boston, 1982, in press.

Feldman, R.G., and Paul, N.M. Identity of emotional triggers in epilepsy. *J. Nerv. Ment. Dis. 162*:345–353, 1976.

Feldman, R.G., and Ricks, N. Nonpharmacologic and behavioral methods, In *Treated of Epilepsy Today*, edited by Ferris, G.S. Medical Economics Company, Oradell, NJ, 1978.

Feldman, R.G., Ricks, N., and Orren, M. Behavioral methods of seizure control. In *Epilepsy: Diagnosis and Management*, edited by Browne, T.R., and Feldman, R.G. Little, Brown, Boston, 1982, in press.

Gladwell, S.R.F., Kaufman, K.R., and Driver, M.V. Psychosis or epilepsy? Differentiation in a complex case. *Dev. Med. Child. Neurol.* 21:95, 1979.

Ives, J.R., Thompson, C.J., and Woods, J.F. Acquisition by telemetre and computer analysis of 4-channel long-term EEG recordings from patients subject to "petit mal" absence attacks. *Electroencephalogr. Clin. Neurophysiol.* 34:665, 1973.

Penry, J.K., Porter, R.J., and Dreifuss, F.E. Simultaneous recording of absence seizures with videotape and electroencephalography: A study of 374 seizures in 48 patients. *Brain* 98:427, 1975.

Porter, R.J., Wolf, A.A., and Penry, J.K. Human electroencephalographic telemetry. *Am. J. EEG Technol.* 11:145, 1971.

Ramani, S.V., Quesney, L.F., Olson, D., and Gumnit, R.J. Diagnosis of hysterical seizures in epileptic patients. *Am. J. Psychiatry* 137:705, 1980.

Slater, E., Beard, A.W., and Githerie, E. The schizophreniform-like psychosis of epilepsy. *Br. J. Psychiatry* 109:95, 1964.

SECTION 3 PSYCHIATRIC ASPECTS

Chapter 8 # Psychiatric Concepts, Definitions and Diagnosis of Hysterical Seizures

ALEC ROY, M.B., B.Chir.(Cantab), D.P.M., M.Phil., M.R.C.P., M.R.C. Psych., F.R.C.P.(C.)

CONCEPTS OF HYSTERIA

Hysteria has fascinated physicians for more than 3000 years and this is well chronicled in Veith's book *Hysteria, The History of a Disease* (1956). Mai and Merskey (1980) have translated Briquet's (1859) monograph *Traité de l'Hysterie* and believe that Briquet's major contribution was to destroy hysteria's historic association with the uterus. Briquet wrote:

> In reviewing the various groups of agents causing hysteria, one must ask with surprise how it was possible over the centuries for the genital organs to be considered so important in the production of this disease. It is easy to see by examining the facts that hysterical neurosis ordinarily results from three groups of modifying agents: emotional suffering, physical suffering and general weakness of the organism.

Among 591 cases of hysteria, Briquet found that the commonest precipitating causes—occurring in 25%—were marital and family problems, "most commonly loss of a husband or close relative or ill treatment of the wife or children" (Mai and Merskey, 1980).

Freud became interested in "hysteria" in Vienna through his association with Breuer and the case of Anna O. and other hysterics. He went to Paris in 1885 to work with Charcot at the Salpetriere. Charcot's dominant interest at that time was hysteria. Charcot demonstrated that hysterical symptoms—seizures, paralysis, sensory changes—could be induced and removed by hypnosis. It was in Paris that Freud received further insight into the fact that the patient's mental life could cause physical symptoms for which there was no organic basis.

Clarke (1980) relates that by 1896 Freud was developing his theories about sexuality and he offers an interesting explanation of the early development of Freud's ideas:

> The first glimmerings of the truth, he (Freud) later wrote, came to him as he was musing over three statements he had heard from his superiors. At one of Charcot's evening receptions, he wrote: I happened to be standing near the great teacher at a moment when he appeared to be telling Brouardel a very interesting story about something that had happened during his day's work. I hardly heard the beginning, but gradually my attention was seized by what he was talking of: a young married couple from a distant country in the East—the woman a severe sufferer (with hysteria), the man either impotent or exceedingly awkward. "Tâchez donc," I heard Charcot repeating, "je vous assure, vous y arriverez." Brouardel, who spoke less loudly, must have expressed his astonishment that symptoms like the wife's could have been produced by such circumstances. For Charcot suddenly broke out with great animation: "Mais, dans des cas pareils c'est toujours la chose génitale, toujours–toujours–toujours," and he crossed his arms over his stomach, hugging himself and jumping up and down on his toes several times in his own characteristically lively way. I know that for a moment I was almost paralyzed with amazement and said to myself: "Well, but if he knows that, why does he never say so?" The second statement, he (Freud) recalled, was when Breuer had said, apparently in reference to the case of an hysteric and the difficulty in discovering the facts: "These things are always secrets d'alcove!"—secrets of the bedchamber. The third statement was by Chrobak who had remarked of one patient that the only realistic hope of cure lay in prescribing regular doses of a normal penis.

In 1908 Freud addressed the subject of hysterical seizures in a paper to the Vienna Psycho-Analytical Society. Freud's (1909) view was that "Investigation of the childhood history of hysterical patients shows that the hysterical attack is designed to take the place of an auto-erotic satisfaction previously practised and since given up." Freud (1909) had views on the determinants of hysterical seizures: "What points the way for the motor discharge of the repressed libido in a hysterical attack is the reflex mechanism of the act of coition—already in ancient times coition was described as 'minor epilepsy.' We might alter this and say that a convulsive hysterical attack is an equivalent of coition."

DEFINITIONS

The recent third edition of the *Diagnostic and Statistical Manual of Mental Disorders, DSM–III* (1980) makes no mention of hysterical neurosis. By using the term "conversion disorder," as below, it implies an unproven mechanism. It does include reference to environmental events as precipitants and to the possible advantages for the patient.

Diagnostic Criteria for Conversion Disorder—DSM-III

1. The predominant disturbance is a loss or alteration of physical functioning, suggesting a physical disorder.
2. Psychological factors are judged to be etiologically involved in the symptom, as evidenced by either:
   a. A temporal relationship between psychologically meaningful environmental stimuli and the initiation or exacerbation of the symptom.
   b. The symptom enables the individual to avoid some activity that is noxious to him.
   c. The symptom enables the individual to get support from the environment that otherwise might not be functioning.
3. Determination that the symptom is not under voluntary control.
4. Failure to explain the symptom by a known physical disorder after appropriate investigation.
5. The symptom is not limited to pain or to a disturbance in sexual functioning.
6. Does not meet the criteria for somatization disorder or schizophrenia.

Hysterical Pseudoseizures

Fenton (1982) discussing problems of nomenclature wrote:

Hysterical pseudoseizures are attacks of sudden unconsciousness usually but not always associated with dramatic motor manifestations, which resemble to a varying degree epileptic seizures. Such attacks have been described by a number of different terms, namely hysteroepilepsy, simulated epilepsy, psychogenic seizures and pseudoseizures. Charcot's term, hysteroepilepsy, implies brain mechanisms in common between epilepsy and hysteria, which do not exist. Simulated epilepsy suggests that the patient is malingering. This is rarely the case since the psychological motivation underlying the seizures is usually unconscious. The term psychogenic seizure is also misleading, as psychogenic factors can play an important role in precipitating frank epileptic attacks. Hence the use of the terms hysteroepilepsy, simulated epilepsy and psychogenic seizures should be avoided. Even the currently most popular term, pseudoseizure, is not ideal, since it implies that the seizure experienced by the patient is not really a seizure! Perhaps pseudoepileptic seizure is a more appropriate term. It acknowledges the occurrence of seizures, their resemblance to genuine epileptic fits and yet avoids the implication of physiological mechanisms in common between epilepsy and hysteria.

Incidence of Hysterical Seizures

Pseudoepileptic seizures are common hysterical syndromes, although their frequency may be declining. Almost three quarters of the hysterics reported by Briquet (1859) had convulsive attacks. Abse (1950) found that hysterical pseudoepileptic seizures were the most common manifestations of hysteria amongst Indian soldiers in the 1940s. Ljungberg (1957) reported 381 patients with hysteria; 20% had hysterical fits, which was the second most common clinical presentation in his series. Reed (1975) reported that 9.1% of the 120 patients discharged from the Maudsley Hospital between 1949 and 1964 with a diagnosis of hysterical neurosis had hysterical fits.

DIAGNOSIS

Past Medical History

The history of the pregnancy and delivery, the birth weight and the presence of any complications should be enquired about, as brain damage may occur at those times. A history of febrile seizures in childhood—especially in the first year of life—is well recognized as implicated in the etiology of mesial temporal sclerosis and the development of later temporal lobe epilepsy (Falconer and Taylor, 1968). A hamartoma should also be considered in those patients with temporal lobe epilepsy.

Organic Brain Disease

In studies of patients with hysteria, associated organic brain disease was found in 60% by Slater (1965), in 63.5% by Whitlock (1967), in 48% by Merskey and Buhrich (1975) and in 40% by Roy (1980). Thus, in considering the differential diagnosis of seizures, the presence of organic brain disease does not in itself favor the diagnosis of epileptic rather than hysterical seizures. Some of these studies may have been biased as they largely came from postgraduate neurological referral centers. Amongst 31 inpatients of a postgraduate psychiatric hospital with a discharge diagnosis meeting strict criteria for hysterical neurosis, only 1 patient had organic brain disease and there was no significant difference between these hysterics and the depressives controls for organic brain disease (Roy, 1979). Referral factors to a non neurological center may be operative here.

A traditional view of hysterical symptom formation has been that since the symptoms are often associated with organic brain disease the latter must be a major determinant of the symptoms. The question is whether the organic brain disease itself or the physical symptoms it produces are the main determinant. To examine this, 34 patients with hysterical seizures were matched with inpatients with depressive neurosis (Roy, 1977). Eleven of the 34 hysterical seizures patients were well-controlled chronic epileptics and they had significantly more organic brain disease than did the controls; they had both organic brain disease and an epileptic seizure to imitate. However, of the 23 hysterical seizures patients without epilepsy, only 2 had organic brain disease as compared with 1 of the depressive controls—not a significant difference. If organic brain disease in itself was the main determinant of hysterical symptoms, the nonepileptic hysterical group should have had significantly more brain disease than the controls; but they did not. This suggests that organic brain disease in itself is not always the major determinant of hysterical symptoms.

Sex and Personality

Briquet was of the opinion "that women are at least 20 times more at risk than men of becoming hysterics." (Mai and Merskey, 1980). Standage (1975) reviewed some of the literature on hysterical seizures (Ferris, 1959; Liske and Forster, 1964) and noted "the relative restriction of such symptoms to young women, and their association with adverse environmental influences and disturbed personality development.... " In a recent study of 22 patients with hysterical seizures, 21 were women (Roy, 1979).

A traditional view has been that hysterics often have a superficial, attention-seeking hysterical personality disorder. However, most experienced clinicians have seen hysterical symptoms in association with diverse personalities. These patients are often assessed as being immature and dependent or as having other personality disorders which make it difficult for them to cope with stress or the inevitable vicissitudes of life. Ramani et al. (1980) reported that none of their epileptics with hysterical seizures had an hysterical personality.

PSYCHIATRIC FACTORS

Freud wrote in 1928: "It is therefore quite right to distinguish between an organic and an 'affective" epilepsy. The practical significance of this is that a person who suffers from the first kind has a disease of the brain, while a person who suffers from the second kind is a neurotic." In a recent study of 50 patients with hysterical neurosis, 32 had hysterical seizures (Roy, 1980). The patients were seen over 3¼ years in 10 London hospitals. All had a psychiatric interview including the Hamilton scale for depression and were asked to complete three questionnaires measuring depressive and anxiety symptoms. When the majority of these patients with hysterical neurosis had been evaluated, it was observed that the majority were depressed. Thus, each was matched for age and sex with the next psychiatric outpatient suffering from depressive neurosis. When the 44 hysterical patients with affective symptoms were compared with the depressive neurosis controls, there were no significant differences on the scores for depressive and anxiety symptoms. The only symptom difference between the hysterics and the depressives was the possession by the hysterics of the hysterical symptom. The hysterical seizure could thus be viewed as a "signal of distress." The six hysterics without depressive symptoms were chronic cases whose condition had lasted over a year. Two had depressive symptoms at the onset of their condition.

Briquet's precipitating causes are severe life events. In recent years Paykel et al. (1969, 1971) and Brown and Harris (1978) have demonstrated the part that adverse life events and chronic difficulties play in the precipitation of neurotic depression. If acute hysteria is similar to acute reactive depression, what are the determinants of the hysterical symptom—the "signal of distress"? Roy (1979) suggested that the major determinant of hysterical symptoms is personal knowledge of a physical symptom. This knowledge may exist because of past or current physical illness in the patient or in a relative or friend. Hysterics would seem to be patients who when in distress and depressed are unable to verbalize this distress. They are unable to seek help in the appropriate manner from those around them or from the medical profession. Instead they adopt what has been called by Parsons "the sick role" and present, or are taken to doctors, with a physical symptom as a "signal of distress." Personal knowledge of a physical symptom probably has its effect through the psychological mechanism of identification—thus epileptics develop hysterical fits. Briquet writing about hysterical seizures expressed a similiar view:

> It is sufficient for one of these patients to see just once a gesture, perceive an action that has shocked them, for them to involuntarily imitate it either in the seizure or in the hysterical symptoms they show at other times ... hysterics have, because of this faculty of imitation, a great influence on each other; ... in my wards, the patient who has the strongest seizures gives the tone to the others.

Amongst the nonepileptic patients with hysterical seizures (Roy, 1980), one began to have her seizures after witnessing and receiving a course of electroconvulsive treatment (ECT) and another claimed to have witnessed a delivery man have an epileptic seizure on her doorstep just before her seizures began. In a study of known chronic epileptics with hysterical seizures, the nature of the hysterical fits closely resembled the type of epileptic fit the patient had (Roy, 1977). Thus, the 5 epileptics with grand mal attacks had convulsion-like hysterical fits. The 4 patients with psychomotor attacks had hysterical fits closer in form to these attacks.

Outpatients with seizures rarely have their seizures witnessed by those with medical training. Nonspecific minor abnormalities in the EEG may be present and may be misreported as suggestive of epilepsy. Such an EEG report may lead to a trial of anticonvulsant medication. This is not an uncommon sequence. Seventeen patients who had been previously diagnosed as epileptic and treated with anticonvulsants were rediagnosed at a later admission as having hysterical seizures only (Roy, 1977). Some of these patients had lived with the diagnosis of epilepsy for years. One patient had become the chairman of the local area epilepsy society, while another had become secretary of her local area epilepsy society. Two other patients, after referral for assessment for temporal lobectomy, were rediagnosed as suffering from hysterical convulsions only. They had been diagnosed elsewhere as suffering from temporal lobe epilepsy which was thought to be refractory to numerous anticonvulsants. Increasing the number or dosage of anticonvulsants may lead to subclinical drug intoxication (as evidenced on the EEG and by blood level estimations), which may in itself facilitate further episodes of hysterical dissociation. Gross (1979) reported that of 19 adolescents with diagnosed psychogenic seizures 13 were initially diagnosed incorrectly as having epilepsy and were treated for an average of 15 months with anticonvulsant medication. Toone and Roberts (1979) described 3 patients with hysterical seizures who presented as being in life-threatening crises and were perceived as requiring urgent and intensive treatment due to the misdiagnosis of status epilepticus.

Roy (1979) tested the hypothesis that, as epilepsy is an organic disorder and hysteria is a psychiatric disorder, psychiatric variables should differentiate hysterical seizures from epileptic seizures. Twenty-two consecutive patients were collected who were admitted for investigation of seizures and whose discharge diagnosis was hysterical seizures only. They were matched with the next patient similarly admitted for investigation of seizures whose discharge diagnosis was epilepsy. All the patients were given a psychiatric interview, including the Hamilton scale for depression, and completed the General Health Questionnaire (30-item version), the Morbid Anxiety and the Wakefield Depression inventories. Significant differences were found between the two groups on five psychiatric variables: a family history of psychiatric disorder, a personal past history of psychiatric disorder, an attempt at suicide, sexual maladjustment (unconsummated marriage, frigidity or promiscuity) and a current depressive syndrome (Table 8.1).

Some confirmation of these findings has come from Stewart et al.

Table 8.1
Psychiatric Background Factors and Mean Scores of Current Affective Symptoms

	Hysterical Seizures ($n = 22$)	Epileptic ($n = 22$)	Significance
Family history of psychiatric disorders	6	1	$P < 0.05$
Past history of psychiatric disorder	20	3	$P < 0.001$
Attempted suicide	14	4	$P < 0.01$
Sexual maladjustment	9	3	$P < 0.05$
General Health Questionnaire (30-item version	17.4	6.2	$P < 0.001$
Hamilton Rating Scale for depression	15.7	4.8	$P < 0.001$
Wakefield Self-Assessment of Depression Inventory	19.8	11.9	$P < 0.001$
Morbid Anxiety Inventory	28.5	17.5	$P < 0.001$
Clinical diagnosis of current affective syndrome	19	6	$P < 0.001$

(1981). Thirty-seven patients with seizure disorders were studied and divided into three groups: 1) patients with organic (neurogenic) seizures alone, 2) patients who exhibited both neurogenic and psychogenic ("hysterical") seizures, and 3) patients with pure psychogenic ("hysterical") seizures. The three groups were compared as to the severity of psychopathology and personality organization. Patients with both mixed and psychogenic seizures had more severe psychopathology. The most common DSM–III diagnoses in the latter two groups were major affective disorders, antisocial personality, borderline personality, and Briquet's syndrome. Patients with psychogenic seizures also had a significantly higher incidence of suicide attempts and past history of psychiatric treatment.

The practical implication of these findings is that if a patient presents as an outpatient complaining of having seizures and these psychiatric variables are present the index of suspicion that these may be hysterical seizures should rise. In such a case, it may be best to admit the patient to the hospital for observation and investigation of the seizures before initiating treatment. This may prevent the misdiagnosis of epilepsy in an outpatient and the initiation of anticonvulsant therapy.

Hysterical Seizures in Epileptics

Similar psychiatric background features were also found when known chronic epileptics with current hysterical symptoms were studied (Table 8.2). In 9 of 10 such patients, their dominant complaint and

Table 8.2
Psychiatric Background Factors

	Epileptic with Hysteria ($n = 10$)	Epileptic Alone ($n = 10$)	Significance
Family history of psychiatric disorder	5	2	n.s.
Past history of psychiatric disorder	10	3	$P < 0.01$
Attempted suicide	8	2	$P < 0.05$
Sexual maladjustment	7	1	$P < 0.01$
Hamilton Rating Scale for depression	21.4	4.1	$P < 0.01$
Wakefield Self-Assessment of Depression Inventory	18.6	11.1	$P < 0.05$
Clinical diagnosis of affective syndrome	10	1	$P < 0.01$

major symptom was hysterical fits which were thought to account for over three quarters of their current attacks. This hysteroepileptic group also differed from a control group of epileptics by more past history of psychiatric disorder, attempted suicide, sexual maladjustment, and current affective syndrome (Roy, 1977). Stewart et al. (1981) found similar results. Thus, these psychiatric factors may also be helpful when the differential diagnosis of current seizures in known chronic epileptics lies between hysterical fits and epilepsy. They suggest that such a patient with an apparent exacerbation of seizures should be considered for admission to the hospital for further observation and investigation.

The occurrence of hysterical seizures in known epileptics is not uncommon. Ramani et al. (1980) in reporting 9 epileptic inpatients admitted with hysterical seizures discussed the not infrequent limitations of clinical criteria for definitive inpatient diagnosis and recommended the usefulness of simultaneous video-EEG monitoring in such situations.

Features of the Seizures

Points in the history usually described as helpful in the differential diagnosis of hysterical seizures from epilepsy are shown in Table 8.3. However, none of these features is totally reliable. For example, patients with hysterical seizures may report that they have had seizures when alone, that they have bitten their tongue in an attack, may have been incontinent of urine and even hurt or bruised themselves during their hysterical seizures. Freud (1909) was aware of these difficulties:

> The involuntary passing of urine is certainly not to be regarded as incompatible with the diagnosis of a hysterical attack ... moreover, biting the tongue may also be met with in undoubted cases of hysteria.... It

Table 8.3
Main Characteristics of Epileptic Fits and Hysterical Attacks*

	Epilepsy	Hysteria
Attack pattern	Similar	Variable
Apparent cause	Absent	Emotional disturbance
Frequency	Rarely more than one a day, except petit mal	Often, frequent, many a day
Others present?	Sometimes when alone; can be nocturnal	Only when other people present (often relatives or consorts) Rarely nocturnal
Where?	Anywhere	Indoors, usually at home
Warning	If present, often stereotyped	Variable, sometimes overbreathing
Onset	Commonly sudden	Often gradual
Scream	At onset	During attack
Convulsion	Stereotyped tonic-clonic phase	Variable, rigidity with random struggling movement
Biting	Tongue	Of lips, hands and other people
Micturition	Very common	Very rarely (*not* never)
Injury	Fairly frequently	Infrequently (*not* never)
Talking during attack	Never	Frequently
Duration	A few minutes	Many minutes, but sometimes much longer
EEG	Abnormal during and between fits	Normal during and between attacks

* Based on Gowers, 1885.
First published by D. F. Scott, in Psychiatric aspects of epilepsy. *Br. J. Psychiatry*, 132: 417–430, 1978. (Reprinted by permission of Dr. Scott and editor *Br. J. Psychiatry*.)

occurs more readily in attacks if the patient's attention had been drawn by the doctor's questions to the difficulties of making a differential diagnosis. Self-injuring may occur in hysterical attacks (more frequently in the case of men). . . .

Drug Reduction

Patients who have hysterical seizures for any length of time are often taking more than one anticonvulsant drug and may also be taking a minor tranquilizer, a major tranquilizer, an hypnotic and, in some instances, an antidepressant. They may be reluctant to see reduction in their anticonvulsant medication for fear that their seizures will exacerbate. However, if it is explained to them that "medication suppresses the signs of different types of attacks in the EEG" there is usually little resistance to the acceptance of slow serial reduction and termination of all medication. This is usually best done by each week reducing the dosage of one drug at a time. This should be accompanied by serial EEGs, including sphenoidal or pharyngeal leads if there is any suspicion of temporal lobe epilepsy. While these investigations are going on, the patient may have a seizure on the ward which can be observed by the nursing staff and the patient can be examined by any available medical staff. If possible the patient should have an EEG after the seizure to look for the presence of postictal slowing on the EEG. In a chronic epileptic patient whose current exacerbation of seizures are pseudo-epileptic, there may come a time during the serial drug reduction that he has a genuine epileptic seizure. It may then be necessary to prescribe an anticonvulsant; one should strive to manage the epilepsy with one anticonvulsant (Shorvon and Reynolds, 1979).

The Psychiatrist

Once a patient has been admitted, the final assessment about the nature of the seizures should include a psychiatric assessment to diagnose hysteria: both negative and positive features must be present. There must be no physical disorder present that is responsible for the current symptoms. The psychiatrist will look for evidence of stress in the patient's life, personality dependency, immaturity, deficiency or vulnerability in order to explain the development of the hysterical reaction. A telephone call to the patient's general practitioner will often be invaluable. He may well have known both the patient and the family over a period of time and have knowledge of chronic or current difficulties. Thus, a psychiatric assessment should be available before the neurological team makes a final diagnosis of hysterical seizures.

The Psychologist

Psychological tests, like the WAIS, should routinely be performed in order to measure intelligence and to see if there are any suggestions of brain damage—as suggested, for example, by a discrepancy between the performance and verbal IQ scores. If organic brain damage is suggested, other psychological tests may be helpful in its localization. The Benton Visual Retention, the Visual Motor Bender-Gestalt, and the Wechsler Memory Test are some of the tests of proven reliability and validity.

The Social Worker

Interviews with key family members or emotionally significant others by the social worker may lead to the discovery of information pertinent to the personality, life situation, and emotional life of the patient, allowing a more complete formulation of why the patient has developed hysterical seizures at this time.

OTHER DIAGNOSTIC AIDS

Working from the observation in animals that electrochemical stimulation of the medial basal hypothalamus increases prolactin release, Trimble (1978) established baseline blood levels of prolactin and again 20 minutes after a clinical fit in 9 epileptics, 11 patients receiving electroconvulsive treatment (ECT) and 7 patients with hysterical seizures. The serum prolactin level rose substantially in the epileptic and ECT groups but not in the hysterics. Trimble concluded that "when the prolactin concentration is above 1000 μ/ml, in the absence of other causes such as high baseline level or medication (phenothiazine), the attack is epileptic rather than hysterical." Levine and Ramirez (1980) recently reported as an aid to differential diagnosis the rapid cessation of pseudoseizures in 3 patients when an ampoule of ammonia was administered. Within a breath or two of the ammonia, the pseudoseizures were aborted.

References

Abse, D. *The Diagnosis of Hysteria.* J. Wright and Sons, Bristol, 1950.
Briquet, P. *Traité de l' Hystérie.* J.B. Balliere et Fils, Paris, 1859.
Brown, G., and Harris, T. *Social Origins of Depression.* Tavistock, London, 1978.
Clark, R.W. *Freud: The Man and the Cause.* Random House, New York, 1980.
Falconer, M., and Taylor, D. Surgical treatment of drug resistant epilepsy due to mesial temporal sclerosis: Aetiology and significance. *Arch. Neurol.* 19:353–361, 1968.
Ferris, G. The recognition of non-epileptic seizures. *South. Med. J.* 52:1557–1567, 1959.
Fenton, G. Hysterical alterations of consciousness. In *Hysteria,* edited by Roy, A. John Wiley, New York, 1982.
Freud, S. (1909). Some general remarks on hysterical attacks. In *The Standard Edition of the Complete Psychological Works of Sigmund Freud,* vol IX, edited by Strachey, J. London, The Hogarth Press, 1959.
Freud, S. (1928). Doestoevsky and parricide. In *The Standard Edition of the Complete Psychological Works of Sigmund Freud,* vol XXI, edited by Strachey, J. London, The Hogarth Press, 1961.
Gross, M. Pseudoepilepsy: A study in adolescent hysteria. *Am. J. Psychiatry* 136:210–213, 1979.
Levine, W., and Ramirez, C. Identifying pseudoseizures with anhydrous ammonia (letter). *Am. J. Psychiatry* 137:995, 1980.
Liske, E., and Forster, F. Pseudoseizures: A problem in the diagnosis and management of epileptic patients. *Neurology* 14:41–49, 1964.
Ljunberg, L. Hysteria: A clinical, prognostic and genetic study. *Acta Psychiatr. Neurol. Scand. Suppl 112,* 1957.

Lowall, J. Psychiatric presentation of seizure disorders. *Am. J. Psychiatry 133:*321–323, 1976.

Mai, F., and Merskey, H. Briquet's treatise on hysteria: A synopsis and commentary. *Arch. Gen. Psychiatry 37:*1401–1405, 1980.

Mai, F., and Merskey, H. Briquet's concept of hysteria: An historical perspective. *Can. J. Psychiatry 26:*57–63, 1981.

Merskey, H., and Buhrich, N. Hysteria and organic brain disease. *Br. J. Med. Psychol. 48:* 359–366, 1975.

Paykel, E., Myers, J., Dienelt, M., Klerman, G., Lindenthal, J., and Pepper, M. (1969) Life events and depression: A controlled study. *Arch. Gen. Psychiatry 21:*753–760, 1969.

Paykel, E., Prusoff, B., and Uhlenhuth, E. Scaling of life events. *Arch. Gen. Psychiatry 21:* 753–760, 1971.

Ramani, V., Quesney, L., Olson, D., and Gumnit, R. Diagnosis of hysterical seizures in epileptic patients. *Am. J. Psychiatry 137:*705–709, 1980.

Reed, J. L. The diagnosis of "hysteria." *Psychol. Med. 5:*13–17, 1975.

Roy, A. Hysterical fits previously diagnosed as epilepsy. *Psychol. Med. 7:*271–273, 1977.

Roy, A. Cerebral disease and hysteria. *Compr. Psychiatry 6:*607–609, 1978.

Roy, A. Identification and hysterical symptoms. *Br. J. Med. Psychology 50:*317–318, 1977.

Roy, A. Hysterical seizures. *Arch. Neurol. 36:*447, 1979.

Roy, A. Hysteria: A case note study. *Can. J. Psychiatry 24:*157–160, 1979.

Roy, A. Hysteria. *J. Psychosom. Res. 24:*53–56, 1980.

Scott, D.F. Psychiatric aspects of epilepsy. *Br. J. Psychiatry 132:*417–430, 1978.

Slater, E. Diagnosis of "hysteria." *Br. Med. J. 1:*1395–1399, 1965.

Standage, K. The aetiology of hysterical seizures. *Can. Psych. Assoc. J. 20:*67–73, 1975.

Stewart, R., Lovitt, R., and Stewart, M. Hysterical seizures are more than hysteria: A research diagnostic criteria, DSM-III and psychometric analysis. Submitted for publication, 1981.

Toone, B.K., and Roberts, J. Status epilepticus: An uncommon hysterical conversion syndrome. *J. Nerv. Ment. Dis. 167:*548–552, 1979.

Trimble, M. Serum prolactin in epilepsy and hysteria. *Br. Med. J. 2(6153):*1682, 1978.

Whitlock, F. The aetiology of hysteria. *Acta Psychiatr. Scand. 43:*144–162, 1967.

Shorvon, S., and Reynolds, E. Reduction in polypharmacy for epilepsy. *Br. Med. J. 2:*1023–1025, 1979.

Chapter 9

Anticonvulsant Drugs and Hysterical Seizures

MICHAEL TRIMBLE, M.B., B.Sc., M.Phil.,
M.R.C.P., M.R.C. Psych.

One of the earliest reports in the English language of a relationship between anticonvulsant drugs and hysterical seizures was that of Niedermeyer et al. (1970) who described 3 patients with anticonvulsant toxicity with such seizures. Two were female, and one of these was achondroplastic. Two had epilepsy, and unequivocal hysterical seizures with typical 'arc de cercle' were seen in all 3 while they were intoxicated. The drugs implicated were primidone and phenytoin, and decrease of the dosages led to disappearance of the hysterical seizures.

The possibility that anticonvulsant drugs play some role in the onset and genesis of hysterical symptoms thus raises another possible association between hysteria and epilepsy, the relationship of which has been reviewed elsewhere (Trimble, 1981b). In order that the possible role that anticonvulsant drugs play in this connection be better understood, the history of the link needs to be briefly reviewed.

The first author to remark on the association between convulsions and hysteria was probably Hippocrates, who in *Diseases of Women* wrote:

> If a woman suddenly becomes voiceless you will find her legs cold, as well as the knees and hands. And if you then palpate the uterus, it is not in the proper place; her heart palpitates, she gnashes her teeth, there is copious sweat, and all the other features characteristic of those who suffer from the sacred disease, and they do all sorts of unheard of things (Simon, 1978).

Willis, the founder of modern neurology and the first to suggest that it was the brain rather than the uterus which was the seat of hysteria, felt that the cause of convulsions was "the spirits being immediately

148

stirred into inordinate motions" which could arise from "passions such as anger or fear" and lead to epilepsy (Dewhurst, 1980). In that, for him, animal spirits were disturbed in both epileptic and hysterical convulsions, he believed they were connected by a similar pathogenesis.

The discussion regarding the association between epilepsy and hysteria continued throughout the eighteenth and nineteenth centuries, leading to the introduction by the French neurologists of the term "hystero-epilepsy." Within this category of disorders many neurologists accepted "hystèro-epilepsie à crises distincts" in which attacks of epilepsy and hysterical convulsions occurred in the same person; although, others suggested that attacks intermediate between hysteria and epilepsy also existed in their own right ("hystéro-epilepsie á crises combinèes"). Other variations on the theme of hysteroepilepsy were the possibilities that hysteria could develop into epilepsy or that an attack of hysteria developed following an epileptic seizure (Marchand, 1920).

Authors such as Landouzy, Briquet and Charcot felt that hystèro-epilepsy à crises combinèe was in fact hysteria, Charcot introducing and preferring the term "hysteria major" to describe this condition. Such writers, however, as Trousseau and Gowers subscribed to the view that attacks intermediate between hysteria and epilepsy existed, both being manifestations of neurosis.

Freud (Freud and Breuer, 1893–1895) explained such relationships in terms of discharge of affects, which in the form of opisthotonos and clonic movements were a reaction for maximal excitation of the brain which included: "purely physical excitation in epileptic attacks, as well as for the discharge of maximal affects in the shape of more or less epileptoid convulsions (viz., the purely motor part of hysterical attacks)." Bratz introduced the term "affect epilepsy" to describe a group of patients who suffered from typical epileptic attacks but were not really to be defined as having epilepsy in that they were psychopaths, who did not undergo mental deterioration with time, and their attacks occurred episodically, being provoked by external stimuli, particularly emotional stress (Bratz, 1911).

A further advance in conceptualization was taken by Pierce Clarke (1923) who presented a "psychobiologic view" of essential epilepsy, such that "given the epileptic constitution and a sufficient amount of environmental stress, the epileptic career is inaugurated." Writing in an era when ideas about the epileptic personality were prominent, he noted that in many cases of epilepsy no neuropathological disorder was demonstrable and that certain patterns of developmental traits were seen prior to the onset of epilepsy. For him, the fit served as an unconscious gratification for the patient's libido; thus, in both epilepsy and the neuroses, infantile motives and the inadequate development of a person's affects and instincts led to the later development of symptoms. Seeking an even more neurophysiological explanation, Jelliffe and White (1929) considered energy flow within the central nervous system. This could be blocked at several different levels and, depending upon which was involved, different clinical consequences ensued. The epileptic seizure itself was considered as "a flight into unconsciousness" being "a break in the life demand for adaptation or an attempt to escape from an intolerable stimulus whether from within (toxin, tumour) or from without (life situation)."

These ideas have persisted through to the present day and have been discussed at length in the writings of Krapf (1957) and Rabe (1970). It is at this point in the history of ideas regarding hysteria and epilepsy that anticonvulsant drugs assume a significant role. Thus epilepsy and hysteria, the latter especially when presenting as major convulsions, have both been viewed as neuroses, both linked to immaturity in the development of the brain, and both occurring with increased frequency in predisposed individuals, the clinical presentation being dependent on the state of the individual nervous system at the time of the attack. Krapf consolidated these ideas, noting that electroencephalograms are often abnormal in the neuroses and that specifically epileptic electroencephalographic activity is not commonly seen in epilepsy. He also made the point that the electroencephalogram in childhood is markedly different from that in an adult, abnormalities tending to get less as age increases (see Fig. 9.1), suggesting that an abnormal electroencephalogram does not indicate in the first place "the predisposition of the brain to explosive discharges of neuronal energy, but rather to the degree of functional maturity of the central organ." Thus epileptiform dysrhythmias were possibly deficiencies in maturation, and these could stem "from psychogenetic factors just as well as from hereditary predispositions . . . ." For him, therefore, certain "psychologically meaningful seizures frequently appear in somatically predisposed individuals . . . there is sometimes an interrelation even between psychological situations and somatic predispositions which makes it possible for them to strengthen or to determine each other to a considerable extent."

Rabe (1970) noted that many patients with hysteria presenting as fits are misdiagnosed as having epilepsy and are treated with anticonvulsant medication. In addition, like Krapf, he emphasized the EEG abnormalities in such patients, noting how the diagnosis of epilepsy had come to rely very much on EEG information, partly because fits themselves are rarely seen by the physician in charge of the patient. In his clinic the combination of hysterical and epileptic seizures occurred in 1.3% of the population, a figure lower than, for example, the 5% given by Bratz. He

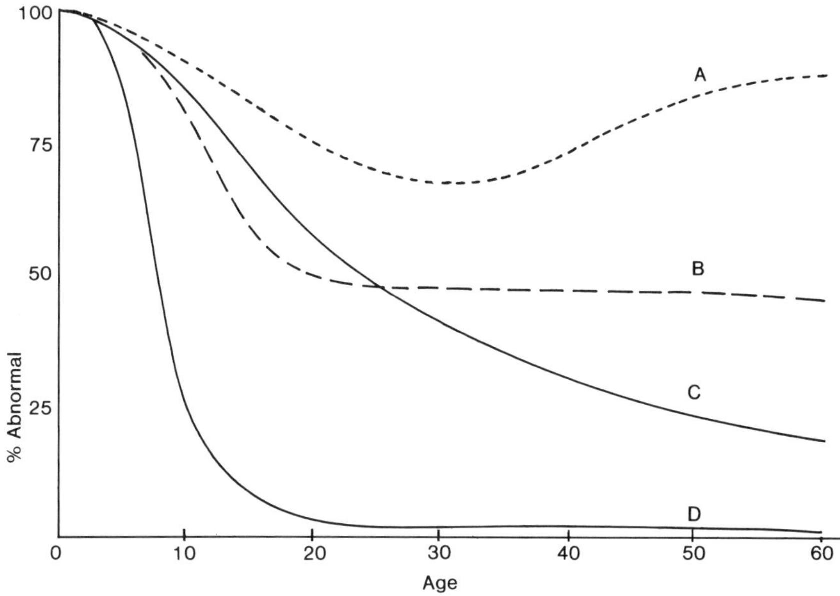

Figure 9.1.   The variation with age of the percentage of cases showing "abnormality" in the EEG. *A*, cerebral tumor (500 cases). *B*, chronic trauma (1200 cases). *C*, idiopathic epilepsy (800 cases). *D*, normal subjects (500). (From D. Hill and G. Parr. *Electroencephalography.* MacDonald & Co., London, 1950, p. 227. Reprinted with permission.)

described 39 patients with combined seizure types, the majority of whom had epilepsy presenting as psychomotor fits with secondary generalization, although 7 had generalized tonic-clonic seizures. He described a number of cases of special interest in which the clinical pattern of the patient's fits changed following treatment, and in particular he discussed cases in which patients appeared to have some switch mechanism triggered by the anticonvulsant therapy. The following case history is typical.

A patient at the age of 10 developed nocturnal grand mal seizures. Twenty years later he developed complex partial epilepsy and was noted to have some "epileptic personality change" and a left temporal spike on the electroencephalogram. Anticonvulsant therapy was initiated and he became fit-free, although he started to complain of hypochondriacal symptoms and lost his appetite. He then began to develop classical hysterical seizures which occurred with great frequency. At this stage the electroencephalogram was normal, the anticonvulsant drugs were withdrawn, the patient started having epileptic fits again, and the hysterical seizures disappeared.

Generally in cases of this type, anticonvulsant medication led to the initiation of hysterical fits and the epileptiform abnormalities on the electroencephalogram tended to disappear. He noted in these patients strong dependence on the family, leading to independence-dependence conflicts, and suggested a psychodynamic explanation such that continuance of fits was necessary for the patient to maintain his dependence on the family. Thus, their suppression by anticonvulsant drugs leads to a disturbance of the patient's psychic equilibrium, being based on unrecognized opposition to freedom from fits.

This "antagonism" between hysterical and epileptic fits outlined by Rabe was also mentioned in the discussion of Niedermeyer's cases and is reminiscent of the ideas introduced earlier by Landolt (1958) with regard to the relationship between schizophreniform psychosis and epilepsy. Thus he described patients with epilepsy who had episodes of psychotic behavior lasting from several days to weeks, during which the electroencephalogram lost its dysrhythmia and was "normalized." When the patient's clinical and mental state returned to normal, the electroencephalographic abnormality was seen to recur. Most of Landolt's patients had focal epilepsy arising from the temporal lobes, and these states could be precipitated by anticonvulsant drugs and terminated by electroconvulsive therapy. Landolt concluded from these studies that there was some form of antagonism between epilepsy and schizophrenia and that the use of anticonvulsant drugs was one mechanism in altering the clinical picture.

Such ideas of antagonism between behavior disorders and epilepsy were, of course, not new. The reciprocal relationship between epilepsy and schizophrenia had been commented on by several authors, and von Meduna introduced convulsive therapy in treatment on the grounds of clinical improvements noted in psychiatric patients following seizures (see Trimble, 1981a).

Rabe, however, implied that it was more than just alteration of the electroencephalogram which led to changes in behavior and hysterical seizures in patients with epilepsy. He suggested that the electroencephalographic disturbances were, in some way, physiological manifestations of a disturbed balance between the ego and the environment. Anticonvulsant drugs therefore do not restore homeostasis to the total system, and the pharmacological suppression of epileptic fits thus only alters the form in which the crises occur (see Fig. 9.2). In this scheme the same pathology therefore underlies both forms of seizures, which are comprehensible only with a knowledge of the psychobiological development of the individual.

In a full review of the literature on hysteria, Merskey (1979) recently confirmed the observations of Niedermeyer that anticonvulsant intoxi-

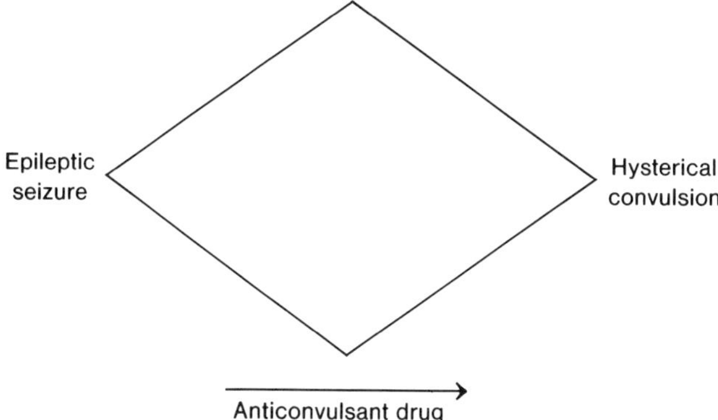

Figure 9.2.   The relationship between epileptic and hysterical convulsions and anticonvulsant drugs.

cation is associated with hysterical symptoms, although he did not provide case illustrations. However, in discussing mechanisms he considered a different means by which anticonvulsant drugs could provoke apparently hysterical seizures, stating: "Many epileptic discharges, especially temporal lobe ones, are so modified in their expression by the use of anticonvulsant medication that they may appear as brief episodes of loss of consciousness, states resembling petit mal and even seemingly hysterical behaviour." In addition he assembled the available data on the relationship between organic brain disease and hysteria and suggested a clear relationship between them. With regard to epilepsy he noted that it was frequently found in samples of patients presenting with hysterical symptoms. In his own series of 89 patients with conversion symptoms, 23 had epilepsy, a higher than expected frequency since 7.2% of inpatients and 14.2% of outpatients had a diagnosis of epilepsy at the hospital where the sample was collected. He also quoted the work of Currie et al. (1971) who followed up 666 patients with temporal lobe epilepsy noting that 17 had a diagnosis of hysteria. Merskey's overall thesis was that cerebral organic disease in some way "neuroticizes" patients, promoting the onset of conversion symptoms. Such a mechanism would, of course, explain the increased incidence of hysteria in epilepsy but would also see anticonvulsant medication as an additional burden to the nervous system and as an additional neuroticizing element.

The evidence that anticonvulsant drugs increase neuroticism is, however, difficult to substantiate. The literature on the relationship between anticonvulsant drugs and disturbances of behavior has been reviewed and indicates that studies in this area are sparse and that the techniques used for the measurement of behavior in most investigations have been inadequate. Many studies were carried out before serum level monitoring was available, and often no attempt was made to distinguish between the effects of anticonvulsant drugs on cognitive abilities, thus impairing performance on psychological tests, as opposed to the effects on behavior which lead to recognizable patterns of psychopathology (Trimble, 1981c). Indeed, there are anecdotal reports of depression occurring as a side effect of phenobarbitone, phenytoin, sulthiame and peganone and of psychoses following phenytoin, primidone, ethosuximide and carbamazepine. They are, however, mainly case reports, although certainly with ethosuximide the onset of a psychosis has been demonstrated to occur with initiation of the drug and with "normalization of the electroencephalogram" during the psychotic episodes.

From the literature reviewed earlier in this chapter, the drugs which would seem most implicated with the induction of hysterical seizures are phenytoin and primidone or phenobarbitone. With regard to the former there are a large number of reports that indicate that phenytoin can impair cognitive abilities, in particular leading to disturbances of visuomotor performance, memory deficits, and possibly impairment of reading abilities, in addition to an insidious deterioration of intellectual function in certain predisposed patients (Trimble, 1981c). Systematic studies of the effects of the drug on behavior are, however, very limited. In low doses in volunteer subjects it has been suggested to have psychotropic properties. Thus Haward (1973), following the demonstration that low doses lead to improved performance in pilots using a flight simulator, referred to the drug as a "normalizer" which raised stress threshold and lowered adrenergic activity when it was high. In order to investigate such effects in more detail, Trimble and Corbett (1980) assessed behavior in 312 epileptic children resident at a hospital school, using standardized and validated rating scales. Each child had a clinical neuropsychiatric examination, and blood was taken for the assessment of serum anticonvulsant levels. The Rutter rating scales were used for the measurement of behavior, which specifically provided estimates of conduct disturbance and neurotic disturbance (Rutter et al., 1970). Fifty percent of the children who were receiving phenobarbitone were rated as having conduct disturbance. While children with neurotic disorder had higher levels of phenytoin than those without, no significant differences were noted in the serum levels of phenobarbitone, phenytoin, primidone or carbamazepine in relation to these disturbances of behavior. Correlation coefficients between serum levels and actual deviant scores for conduct and neurotic disorder likewise failed to demonstrate significant associations between them. It is important to note, however, that in this study very few of the children were intoxicated with their drugs; while not substantiating the hypothesis that anticonvulsant drugs themselves neuroticize patients, it does not negate the original proposition that anticonvulsant drug toxicity, with higher serum levels, may do so.

More recently we have been assessing the relationship between improvements in behavior and alteration of drug therapy in patients with epilepsy and volunteers that has bearing on this problem (Trimble et al., 1981). In one study, volunteers were given either phenytoin, carbamazepine or sodium valproate and their cognitive abilities and mood were assessed in comparison with an equivalent time spent on matched placebo tablets in three crossover design experiments. Not only were different effects of these drugs noted on cognitive function, especially memory, with phenytoin leading to most impairment, but differences in mood were also detected. In particular, subjects on phenytoin rated themselves on a modified mood objective check-list to be more anxious, tired, aggressive and depressed than on placebo; in the carbamazepine experiment, changes were in the opposite direction, suggesting improvement. In another study, 75 patients with epilepsy were given a variety of cognitive tests, including the mood check list, while undergoing changes in drug therapy, testing being carried out before and at 3 and 6 months after the alteration of medication (Thompson, 1981). Of 20 undergoing drug reductions, significant improvements were noted on the majority of cognitive tests used, and a significant fall in anxiety ratings was seen at 6 months, with a trend for improvement in fatigue, aggression and depression. In these patients who were all on polytherapy, the major fall was in phenobarbitone levels, although primidone and sodium valproate levels also declined. Mean phenytoin levels, however, for the group remained unchanged. These data suggest that anticonvulsant drugs do increase psychopathology, especially anxiety, although no drug clearly emerges as being more prone than others to do this. The drug withdrawal study, with improvement in rating scale scores, indicates why some patients with anticonvulsant toxicity and hysterical seizures improve with regulation of their medication to give lower serum levels.

Two other mechanisms of the relationship between hysteria and anticonvulsant drugs should be briefly considered. First, a number of patients present with nonepileptic convulsions who do not have epilepsy (Trimble, 1981b). Thus, while it is often said that hysterical convulsions nearly always occur in patients who have preexisting epilepsy, this is manifestly not true in clinical practice. It is disturbing to note that conservative estimates of the incidence of patients who do not have epilepsy who are attending an epileptic clinic with a diagnosis of epilepsy is in the region of 20% (Jeavons, 1977). Such people, for the reasons outlined by Rabe (1970), are susceptible to being started on anticonvulsant drugs by physicians and because of their personality may well be prone to the development of dependence upon drugs, in particular to barbiturates. The following case history gives an example of such a presentation:

> C.T., a 32-year-old female, was well until 4 months prior to admission, when she started having episodes of loss of consciousness which were diagnosed as epilepsy and for which she was prescribed phenobarbitone. These were abused and she started taking increased amounts of the drug, leading to an increased frequency of seizures. On admission to hospital she had ataxia, dysarthria and diplopia and was tearful and agitated. She demonstrated repeated attacks of tonic rigidity, with frothing at the mouth and urinary incontinence, sometimes leading to opisthotonic posturing. The phenobarbitone serum level was 198 μmol/liter and the phenytoin level was 81 μmol/liter. Further history taking revealed early neurotic traits, a long history of abnormal illness behavior and hospitalizations, and current interpersonal stresses, especially within her marriage. On the day she had her first "attack," her husband had been arrested on a felony charge. Following reduction of the anticonvulsants and readjustment of her therapy with recognition of the florid psychopathology, the seizures abated and have not returned.

In this situation, therefore, a nonepileptic patient with elements of the hysterical personality was started on barbiturates. When these were withdrawn a major tonic-clonic convulsion ensued, thus substantiating for the treating physician a diagnosis of epilepsy and leading to continued misadministration of anticonvulsant drugs with resultant toxicity and further symptoms of hysteria.

The second alternative is that patients with or without epilepsy may be prescribed anticonvulsant drugs that lead to side effects other than hysterical convulsions but which are mistakenly diagnosed as hysteria. The second case history presented here is an example of this.

> E.F., a 54-year-old female, was admitted to hospital with a 9-year history of seizures, progressive dementia, and loss of balance. Always a solitary person, the patient's attacks first started following the death of her father, and 3 years later when her mother died she, for the first time in her life, started living alone. A diagnosis of epilepsy was made and she was started on phenobarbitone and later was given phenytoin. One year prior to admission she had been taken into a local mental hospital and then had been transferred to an old people's home, with a diagnosis of dementia. On examination she was withdrawn and unkempt, was ataxic and dysarthric, and had persistent tremor of her head and upper limbs. The latter was thought to be hysterical, arising in a patient with either dementia or

schizophrenia. The phenobarbitone level was 272 μmol/l, and the phenytoin level was 90 μmol/l.

On withdrawal of her anticonvulsants she lost many of her signs and symptoms and, following rehabilitation, ceased having seizures and assumed a semi-independent life outside hospital.

In this case, involuntary movements were induced by anticonvulsant intoxication, a side effect now well recognized (Ahmad et al., 1975), which became diagnosed as hysteria. The consequences were nearly disastrous since the patient was institutionalized and would have remained so if not for the intervention of a perceptive physician. The relationship between abnormal movements and hysteria is an interesting and complicated one (Trimble, 1981a), but the point is here emphasized that anticonvulsant drug toxicity can present as a whole range of signs and symptoms, which includes abnormal movements of a variety of types including hysterical seizures per se.

It is hoped that this brief discussion will increase recognition of the relationship between anticonvulsant drugs and hysterical seizures, since, clinically, toxicity with these compounds is still commonly encountered but their role in the production of behavior disturbances in patients is often not considered. The incidence of these problems should diminish with improved management of epilepsy, particularly with the use of serum anticonvulsant level monitoring and the use of newer anticonvulsant drugs such as carbamazepine and sodium valproate, which appear to be less likely to provoke toxicity and behavior disorders than their forerunners.

References

Ahmad, S., Laidlaw, J., Houghton, G.W., and Richens, A. Involuntary movements caused by phenytoin intoxication in epileptic patients. *J. Neurol. Neurosurg. Psychiatry 38*:225–231, 1975.

Bratz, Die affekt epileptischen Anfälle der Neuropathen und Psychopathen. *Monatsschr. Psychiatr. Neurol. 29*:45, 1911.

Currie, S., Heathfield, K.W.G., Henson, R.A., and Scott, D.F. Clinical course and prognosis of temporal lobe epilepsy. *Brain 94*:173–190, 1971.

Dewhurst, K. *Thomas Willis' Oxford Lectures.* Sandford Publications, Oxford, 1980.

Freud, S., and Breuer, J. (1893–1895) *Studies on Hysteria.* Penguin Books Ltd., Middlesex, 1974.

Haward, L. Effects of D.P.H. upon concentration in pilots. *Riv. Med. Aeronaut. Spaz. 12*: 372–374, 1973.

Hill, D., and Parr, G. *Electroencephalography.* MacDonald & Co., London, 1950.

Jeavons, P.M. Choice of drug therapy in epilepsy. *Practitioner 219*:542–556, 1977.

Jelliffe, S.E., and White, W.A. *Diseases of the Nervous System.* H.K. Lewis, London, 1929.

Krapf, E.E. On the pathogenesis of epileptic and hysterical seizures. *Bull. W.H.O. 16*:749–762, 1957.

Landolt, H. Serial encephalographic investigations during psychotic episodes in epileptic patients and during schizophrenic attacks. In *Lectures on Epilepsy*, edited by Lorenz de Haas. Elsevier, London, 1958, pp. 91–133.

Marchand, L. *Epilepsie et Hystéria*. La Press Médicale, 1920, pp. 627–628.

Merskey, H. *The Analysis of Hysteria*. Baillière Tindall, London, 1979.

Neidermeyer, E., Blumer, D., Holscher, E., and Walker, B.A. Classical hysterical seizures facilitated by anticonvulsant toxicity. *Psychiatr. Clin.* 3:71–84, 1970.

Pierce Clark, L. The psychobiologic concept of essential epilepsy. *J. Nerv. Ment. Dis.* 57: 433–444, 1923.

Rabe, F. *Die Kombination hysterischer und epileptischer Anfalle*. Springer-Verlag, Berlin, 1970.

Rutter, M., Graham, P., and Yule, W. A neuropsychiatric study in childhood. William Heinemann, Philadelphia, 1970.

Simon, B. *Mind and Madness in Ancient Greece*. Cornell University Press, Ithaca, NY, 1978.

Thompson, P. The effects of anticonvulsant drugs in the cognitive functioning of patients with epilepsy and normal volunteers. Ph.D. Thesis, University of London, 1981.

Trimble, M.R., and Corbett, J. Behavioural and cognitive disorders in epileptic children. *J. Irish Med. Assoc.* 73(suppl):21–28, 1980.

Trimble, M. *Neuropsychiatry*. Wiley & Sons, Chichester, 1981a.

Trimble, M.R. Hysteria. In *Psychiatric Aspects of Epilepsy*, edited by Trimble, M.R., and Reynolds, E.H. Churchill Livingstone, New York, 1981b.

Trimble, M.R. Anticonvulsant drugs, behaviour and cognitive abilities. In *Current Developments in Psychopharmacology*, edited by Valzelli, and Essman, W. 1981c.

Trimble, M.R., Thompson, P., and Corbett, J. Anticonvulsant drugs, cognitive function and behaviour. in press, 1981.

Chapter 10 # Management of Hysterical Seizures

ALEC ROY, M.B., B.Chir.(Cantab), D.P.M.,
M.Phil., M.R.C.P., M.R.C. Psych.,
F.R.C.P.(C.)

THE SETTING

The management of patients with hysterical seizures may be difficult. This is due to the already discussed difficulties in diagnosis—involving as it does the interface between neurology, psychiatry and electroencephalography; the personality disturbance that these patients may have; the emotional reactions of the staff; and the vicissitudes of the treatment process. Hospitalization may last several weeks. The ideal situation from the outset is for such patients to be investigated and treated in a neuropsychiatric ward, jointly staffed by neurologists and psychiatrists, where the nursing staff over time manage many such patients and become experienced in the necessary diagnostic and therapeutic skills. However, such settings are rarely found except in a few postgraduate centres. In other circumstances though, successful diagnosis and management can be routinely obtained. However, in this author's view, it is a mistake to simply investigate and diagnose without making appropriate short-term and long-term management plans. Due to pressure for medical and neurological beds, bias and other factors, patients with hysterical seizures are not infrequently investigated, with or without psychiatric consultation, and then discharged. If that course is dictated by events then the patient should, of course, be referred back to the care of the general practitioner with a recommendation that psychiatric treatment should be sought. If seizures are frequent or severe depression is present, the patient should be kept in hospital.

MEDICAL INVESTIGATIONS

Successful psychiatric management of the patient with seizures goes hand in hand with thorough physical examination and investigation (see earlier chapters). As a consequence, the patient feels reassured that his or her presenting problem is being taken seriously. The patient should be seen frequently by the doctor during the hospitalization to talk about the purpose of each investigative procedure and any drug reduction. Anxiety is thus diminished and the patient-doctor rapport is enhanced. Much may depend on the development of this early rapport with the doctor, or one of the team, for later successful management.

ATTITUDES

It is necessary for all staff to always maintain a positive professional attitude. In hospital, once the absence of epilepsy has been suggested in patients with seizures it is unfortunately not uncommon for the patient to be called "malingering," "hysterical" or "an hysteric" by members of the nursing or medical staff. The patient invariably perceives any negative attitudes of her nurses or doctors and successful management is then compromised and made more difficult. This is partly because the patient may have no or only limited insight into the fact that the convulsions are due to emotional problems, and she may become further distressed by inferences or statements that she is "putting it on," "acting," "hysterical" or "could stop it if she wished." The patient is then placed in a dilemma. Even when the insight that her seizures are due to "nerves," is gained, it is difficult for the patient to seek or accept help from staff and doctors that she has sensed are rejecting, hostile, critical or who have other negative attitudes toward her. However, if the staff has developed negative attitudes toward the patient, such hostility may become countertherapeutic and transfer to a psychiatric ward may be expedient.

THE TEAM

Often some of these patients' personality difficulties manifest themselves in the hospital. They may want special attention or favors or may want exceptions made for them. They may play one staff member against the other. If frustrated in their demands, they may threaten to harm themselves or may have temper outbursts. Not all patients with pseudoepileptic seizures pose these management problems. But it is always essential for all those treating and involved with the patient—nurses, doctors, social worker, psychologist, occupational therapist—to work as a team. This means multidisciplinary team meetings where information can be communicated and shared, problems discussed and plans formulated. For example, when a degree of certainty exists that the current seizures are hysterical it may be decided that the staff will give no attention to further seizures. It is important for the team members, in the face of vicissitudes in management, to be consistent in their approach to the patient. In general, it is best to be firm about limits.

THE PSYCHIATRIST

The psychiatrist may have seen the patient as part of the assessment. Once the diagnosis of pseudoepileptic seizures has been made, the psychiatrist may be consulted again, if necessary, about appropriate treatment strategies or may be asked to treat the patient himself. If the patient is transferred to a psychiatric ward, the psychiatrist is likely to be the leader of the multidisciplinary team treating her and will coordinate the work of the other disciplines.

THE SOCIAL WORKER

The social worker often has important social case work and psychotherapeutic roles with such patients. Often patients have financial problems, housing difficulties, employment problems or family conflicts which may be amenable to social case work. Financial help, new living arrangements or the alleviation of interpersonal conflicts may be important therapeutic interventions that the social worker may make in the patient's environment.

It may be helpful to have one or a series of conjoint meetings—for example, between an adolescent girl and her mother, between husband and wife (or cohabitee), or between other family members. Such treatment interventions may be done with the social worker and doctor working together as cotherapists or with the psychiatrist or a psychiatrically trained social worker working alone. Bringing the family into interviews at an appropriate stage of management will often lead to clarification of family dynamics, the expression and ventilation of relevant family conflicts, and may serve to reduce any "secondary gain" that the seizures bring to the patient.

THE PSYCHOLOGIST

In those patients suffering from recurrent or chronic anxiety, it may be helpful to instruct the patient about anxiety-relieving techniques. A psychologist will teach the patient a method of muscular relaxation or a cognitive method of self-control of anxiety. The psychologist may also be involved with behavior therapy for discrete problems discussed later.

In some instances the psychologist may be of help to the treating team when it wishes to formulate treatment plans to minimize the gain that may accrue to the patient from her environment in terms of rewards for her "illness behavior" and to maximize and reward normal seizure-free behavior. Kendell (1972), for example, is of the view that an essential element in the treatment of hysteria is to minimize the benefits of illness behavior and to maximize the benefit of well behavior.

MEDICATION

Hypnotics

Medication may be useful in the initial course of treatment. Often those patients who are anxious or depressed have difficulty in getting to sleep and have disturbed sleep or early morning waking. Sleep disturbance may be accentuated due to admission to a hospital ward. A mild hypnotic may be helpful and a good night's sleep may be very refreshing, especially for the patient who lies awake worrying and ruminating about the past or about current conflicted unhappy relationships or other difficulties.

Anxiolytics

The management of anxiety is a common problem with these patients. These are often patients with chronically anxious personalities who become very anxious before admission, and anxiety may exacerbate and become an acute problem while the patient is trying to cope with the new conscious knowledge that the seizures may be due to "nerves." If the patient is not already receiving anxiolytics before admission, antianxiety drugs are best avoided, if possible, as dependency on such medication may lead to later vicissitudes in management. Often patients are already taking tranquilizers prescribed by previous doctors or their general practitioner. If the dosage is not excessive, it may be best to allow the patient to continue taking these while she tries to cope with the new knowledge about the cause of her seizures. Toward the end of the hospital stay, previously prescribed anxiolytic drugs should be gradually withdrawn. For example, if the patient is taking a total of 15 mg of valium each day, a schedule of withdrawal of 5 mg a week agreed with the patient is likely to succeed. This reduction schedule can, if necessary, be continued on an outpatient basis. For the not infrequent patient who is taking substantially larger daily doses of valium, more cautious withdrawal of 2 mg every few days is indicated in order to prevent withdrawal seizures. These seizures are not uncommon in patients taking large daily doses of valium and clearly are an unfortunate occurrence in a patient in whom the absence of seizures is a goal of management. Many such patients are reluctant to give up their tranquilizers. Education of the patient about dependence on anxiolytics and their loss of efficacy due to tolerance may help to prevent resistance from the patient and thus lessen conflict with her doctor.

Antidepressants

Symptoms of depression are usually present to some degree and often a depressive syndrome may be easily diagnosable. The severity of depression may vary from mild to moderately severe to severe. However, severe depression is rare. Admission to hospital may in itself be very helpful in alleviating depression, because the patient is removed from external environmental stresses and conflicted interpersonal relations. At a psychological level, admission may signify to the patient that their "signal of distress" has been perceived by the doctor. Once in hospital, interaction with the nurses, doctors and other patients may also lead to attenuation of depressive symptoms. If a moderately severe depressive state does not resolve within a week or two of admission, antidepressant drugs should be considered. Tricyclic antidepressants should be the drugs of first choice. Compounds like amitriptyline and trimipramine have a sedative side effect and this can be turned to good effect if the total daily dose is taken at night, as any request for additional night hypnotics can be resisted by explaining this sedative side effect to the patient. Although antidepressant drugs must be taken for up to 2 weeks before expecting their specific therapeutic antidepressant effect, the patient may feel significantly better before that as a consequence of suggestion, having a better night's sleep and other nonspecific therapeutic effects. Antidepressant drugs must be prescribed in adequate dosage, which for the tricyclic compounds is usually between 75 and 150 mg daily, and for an adequate time, which should be not less than a month. The side effects of dry mouth, possible initial blurred vision etc. should be explained to the patient. These side effects are often maximal during the first few days of such a course and it is usually best to start with a small dose and gradually increase it. This approach usually leads to better compliance by the patient. In occasional patients, severe depression with intense preoccupation with death or guilt, with marked feelings of hopelessness, worthlessness and suicidal ideation may require a course of electroconvulsive treatment. This decision, however, must be made by a psychiatrist.

PSYCHOTHERAPY

Psychotherapy is usually the main treatment modality with these patients. If the patient has a history of frequent seizures, or seizures at regular intervals, or was admitted as an emergency after an exacerbation of hysterical seizures, she will often comment on the paradox that she has had few or no seizures since coming into hospital, despite reductions that may have been made in her medication. Then, as these patients are not malingerers, usually spontaneously or after gentle questioning the patient will wonder "if it could be my nerves." At such a lead from the patient, the doctor should encourage further reflection and talk about such a possibility. Such open-ended questions as "What do you mean?", "Do you want to say some more about that?", "Why do you think it might be your nerves?", or "Have there been problems or difficulties which have been worrying you recently?" will encourage the patient to start to talk and eventually to confide and trust in her doctor. It goes without saying that blunt statements from the doctor that the staff think the attacks are "hysterical" or "put on" will not encourage doctor-patient rapport. If at this time the doctor enters into a dialogue with the patient, insight into the psychogenic nature and cause of the seizures often quickly increases. It must be stressed that the patient's motives for having hysterical seizures are largely unconscious and hidden from awareness. Talking with the doctor over time will gradually allow such motives to be brought into the patient's awareness and thus from the unconscious to the conscious mind. This is usually accompanied by the termination of seizures or, at least, by a marked reduction in their frequency.

However, this is often a painful process for the patient. She has to cope with the new knowledge she has gained about herself. This is often accompanied by a lowering of self-esteem, and depression may be exacerbated at this time or may develop for the first time. By avoiding confrontation with the patient about the nature of her seizure, she is allowed to adjust gracefully over time and to save face. It must be remembered that she has to temporarily live on the ward and face not only the nurses but also her relatives at visiting time who may well have asked for current progress reports from the nursing staff.

Supportive psychotherapy involves encouraging the patient to talk about difficulties, problems, worries and conflicts and also involves listening and discussing these with her. Psychotherapy usually continues over time. It is important to prevent ambiguity in the patient's mind about this. Therefore, at the outset it is best to state approximately how many sessions there may be, their frequency, how long each session will last, when and where they will take place, and that their purpose is for the patient to discuss her problems and difficulties. It is as well at the outset to mention indirectly the phenomenon called "transference" by saying that it is common that patients, when talking over time to a doctor, often feel both negative and positive feelings toward the doctor, that this is quite normal and may be commented on by the doctor. We now know from psychotherapy research that nonpossessive warmth, nonjudgmental empathy and acceptance are important elements in facilitating both symptom relief and personality change in patients in psychotherapy.

It is helpful in the first psychotherapy sessions to try to set goals for the treatment. These are best decided by the patient and may vary from the objective—like stop having seizures, getting over depression, obtaining a job, leaving home or breaking off a painful relationship—to more subjective areas—such as examining relationship difficulties, dependency needs or needs for attention, or other personality problems. The goals of psychotherapy will vary with the patient. Their attainment will depend on the number of sessions, the patient's life circumstances, her personality strengths and weaknesses, the patient's ability to enter into a therapeutic relationship, her self-reflective capacity, intelligence, age, and motivation for personal change.

Supportive psychotherapy should be a treatment skill possible for the great majority of doctors. Such listening and talking with the patient will probably begin while the patient is in hospital and may continue, after the patient is discharged, in outpatient appointments. Jerome Frank's book *Persuasion and Healing* (1961) is perhaps the most useful introduction to such psychotherapy. The instillation of hope in the patient is of great importance. If a psychiatrist is liasing with the medical service, it may be best to refer the patient to him because of his training, knowledge and experience in treating psychiatric patients and his experience in the techniques of psychotherapy. For those patients who have had their hysterical seizures for more than a few days or weeks, the value of supportive psychotherapy by one doctor over time cannot be overstated. Support by one doctor over time will usually allow the giving up of seizures as a "signal of distress" while a better adjustment is encouraged and achieved.

In his 1909 paper on hysterical seizures, Freud wrote of "the service of the secondary purposes, with which the illness allies itself, as soon as, by producing an attack, the patient can achieve an aim that is useful to him. In the last case the attack is directed at particular individuals; it can be put off till they are present and it gives an impression of being consciously simulated." Freud's general editor James Strachey (1959) states that "this seems to be the first appearance of the actual term 'flight into illness'." These issues, particularly the "aim" of the attacks or the persons against whom they are directed, may emerge during the assessment or later in psychotherapy and may become the focus for extensive reflection and discussion.

MARITAL THERAPY

Many patients with hysteria are married or cohabiting. In Roy's (1980) study, 30 of the 50 hysteria patients were married or cohabiting. Similarly amongst 22 hysterical seizure patients, 21 were women and many were married (Roy, 1979). It was the strong clinical impression in those studies that often the hysterical syndrome was a "signal of distress" about a severe marital problem.

Resolution of marital conflict and distress by marital therapy may prove to be a very important therapeutic intervention in such patients. Careful assessment is needed as to the nature of the marital problems, their causes, and whether both marital partners are prepared to be seen together and are motivated to seek changes in their relationship. Confidentiality may complicate the issues. For example, a wife may eventually reveal to her doctor that she knows that her husband is having an affair. The husband, however, may be unaware of his wife's knowledge of this. Or the wife herself may be having an affair.

There are several types of marital therapy. Broadly speaking the two main schools of marital therapy are psychodynamic and behavioral. This subject has been well reviewed by Crown (1976). Crowe (1973) carried out a study in which psychodynamic and behavioral marital therapy were compared and reported that patients receiving behavioral marital therapy had a better outcome. The treatment team may not be experienced in marital treatment or may not wish to treat marital problems. In such situations, referral to a marital counseling agency may be considered.

BEHAVIORAL PSYCHOTHERAPY

Apart from the talking psychotherapies, behavioral psychotherapy may be useful for some of these patients. For example, immature, dependent and unassertive individuals lacking social skills may benefit from social skills training. Those who have difficulty asserting themselves may benefit from assertiveness training. Patients with sexual problems may require behavioral treatment. This may be treatment for vaginismus or anorgasmia in the women and treatment for impotence or premature ejaculation in the men. Clearly in married patients, or those with a regular sexual partner, this can be of great benefit. In the occasional patient with associated agoraphobia, social phobias or other phobias, assessment for a behavior therapy intervention may be very useful.

GROUP PSYCHOTHERAPY

The psychiatrist may decide that certain patients with personality difficulties may benefit from group psychotherapy with other psychiatric outpatients with similar problems. This may be beneficial in terms of personal insight, from the comments of others in the group, and in terms of offering a group where the patient may learn to improve her interpersonal communication skills.

VOCATIONAL REHABILITATION

Referral to a vocational assessment, counseling and rehabilitation service may prove an invaluable adjuvant to treatment in some patients. This is because many pseudoseizure patients either are unemployed or, if working, are dissatisfied with their occupational level or have interpersonal clashes with supervisors and co-workers. Lack of work, lack of work skills and maladjustment at work are all aspects of the patient's life in which helpful intervention may have a positive effect on both the resolution of current problems and on the longer term psychiatric and social adjustment and prognosis.

The initial step is referral of a patient with such difficulties to a vocational rehabilitation service. Usually an intake interview with a trained vocational rehabilitation worker occurs during which the educational and occupational record, skills and future aspirations of the patient are determined. If necessary and helpful for complete assessment, further interviews may be arranged to allow for intelligence, aptitude, skills and psychological testing. Eventual recommendations may vary from simple counseling about how and where to best look for appropriate work to placement in a work adjustment program, which may be helpful for those who have had interpersonal difficulties at work, to recommendations to funding agencies for educational skills upgrading or skills training programs for certain selected patients.

FOLLOW-UP

At the end of the admission it is important for one member of the team, usually the doctor, to liase with the follow-up therapists, agencies and the general practitioner and for the appropriate typed reports to be sent out. This may also serve to prevent readmission elsewhere, where the fact of an earlier admission to a previous hospital may not initially be known, and thus prevent reinvestigation and possibly the reintroduction of anticonvulsants.

There have been few detailed follow-up studies of patients with hysterical seizures. Kraepelin (1913) wrote that patients with hysterical seizures had a good prognosis. Ljungberg (1957), as part of a larger follow-up study of patients with hysteria, reported that 42% of those with hysterical seizures still had hysterical seizures at follow-up 5 years later and had a significantly less favorable outcome than did patients with astasia-abasia. Clinical experience would suggest that the prognosis both in psychiatric and social terms is variable. For example, an 18-year-old employed girl, who is immature and dependent, who has her first psychiatric episode when she presents with a series of hysterical seizures when her first serious boyfriend breaks off with her probably has a better prognosis than does the 23-year-old unemployed, personality disordered, lesbian drug abuser who has a long history of maladjustment, overdoses, recurrent depression, interpersonal crises and psychiatric admissions. Common sense suggests that early psychiatric intervention and continued psychiatric supervision, where indicated, may help to ensure a better prognosis. Fenton (1982), who has had extensive personal experience in the management of patients with pseudoseizures, is of the view "that most have a favourable outcome, though some may continue to respond at times of stress with occasional clusters of pseudoseizures." However, further follow-up data are needed as to the natural history of the condition and as to the best treatment interventions.

References

Crowe, M. Conjoint marital therapy: Advice or interpretation. *J. Psychosom. Res.* 17:309–315, 1973.

Crown, S. Marital breakdown: Epidemiology and psychotherapy. In *Recent Advances in Clinical Psychiatry*, edited by Grossman, G. Churchill Livingstone, New York, pp. 200–226, 1976.

Fenton, G. Hysterical alterations of consciousness. In *Hysteria*, edited by Roy, A. John Wiley, New York, 1982.

Frank, J. *Persuasion and Healing.* Johns Hopkins Press, Baltimore, 1961.

Freud, S. (1909). Some general remarks on hysterical attacks. In *The Standard Edition of the Complete Psychological Works of Sigmund Freud*, vol. IX, General Editor, James Strachey. The Hogarth Press, London, 1959.

Kendell, R. A new look at hysteria. *Medicine* 30:1780–1782, 1972.

Kraepelin, E. Uber Hysterie. *Z. Neurol. Psychiatr.* 18:261, 1913.

Ljungberg, L. Hysteria: A clinical, prognostic and genetic study. *Acta Psychiatr. Neurol. Scand.* Supplement 112, 1957.

Roy, A. Hysterical seizures. *Arch. Neurol. 36:*447, 1979.

Roy, A. Hysteria. *J. Psychosom. Res.* 24:53–56, 1980.

Strachey, J. Footnote I., p. 232. In *The Standard Edition of the Complete Psychological Works of Sigmund Freud*, vol. IX. The Hogarth Press, London, 1959.

 # Psychogenic Seizures in Childhood and Adolescence

DANIEL T. WILLIAMS, M.D.
DAVID I. MOSTOFSKY, Ph.D.

The impact of a seizure in any individual's life experience is usually quite dramatic, whether the cause of the seizure be purely neurogenic, purely psychogenic or some combination thereof. The impact of this event is all the more accentuated in the life of a child or adolescent, whose coping resources are generally more limited than those of the adult. This chapter will address some of the special considerations which apply to the genesis, diagnosis and treatment of psychogenic seizures in childhood and adolescence.

Epidemiological studies have indicated that the incidence of epilepsy is highest in the age-group under 5 years (152/100,000) and is lowest between the ages of 20 and 70 years (40/100,000) (Glaser, 1979). Furthermore, there are two peaks in the curve of the onset of seizures. The first peak is in the first 2 years of life and the second is at the age of puberty. Thus, it is clear that children and adolescents merit special attention with regard to developmental issues that color the psychiatric complications of epilepsy and the psychogenic imitations thereof in the form of pseudoseizures. Comparable epidemiological data are not currently available regarding the incidence of psychogenic seizures in these younger age-groups. However, clinical experience of those working closely with seizure patients suggests that pseudoseizures and psychogenically precipitated neurogenic seizures are encountered with significant frequency. It follows that an understanding of their clinical features and appropriate treatment strategies should be part of the repertoire of pediatric neurologists and mental health practitioners working in this area.

COGNITIVE ISSUES

Since epilepsy occurs with relative frequency in patients with documented organic brain lesions and since epilepsy itself connotes brain dysfunction, it is clear that seizure patients are at substantial risk for the associated cognitive impairments that often accompany such brain dysfunction, including mental retardation, learning disabilities, and attention deficit disorders (Cantwell, 1977; Shaffer, 1977). These limitations, which by definition put the seizure patient at a competitive disadvantage with nonepileptic siblings and peers, predispose to the development of secondary psychopathology, including a variety of emotional and behavioral disorders as well as pseudoseizures. In a similar vein, youngsters who have various forms of cognitive impairment but who do not have a true neurogenic seizure disorder may be exposed, by virtue of a special class of institutional placement, to those who do have neurogenic seizures. The awareness of the special attention and treatment afforded to seizure patients may then generate strong incentives either consciously or unconsciously for the development of pseudoseizures and the associated secondary gain which they engender.

EMOTIONAL ISSUES

A central psychological correlate of the loss of consciousness associated with most seizures is the sense of loss of control which is involved. This immediately creates a circumstance of helplessness and dependence in the patient and thrusts the family and others into a more supportive role. For children and adolescents, who under the best of circumstances are struggling with great ambivalence regarding the process of separation and individuation from parents and parent surrogates, the presence of seizures may generate a great regressive pull in the youngsters' relationships with parents and other authority figures (Williams et al., 1978). The hovering presence of parents or others monitoring anticonvulsant medication, often limiting physical activities and bringing the youngster to many medical appointments contributes to the generation of a special status for the seizure patient. There may be a great yearning in some seizure patients to augment this status at times of stress. There seems to be a similar yearning that leads pure pseudoseizure patients to attain this status when they feel threatened or overwhelmed.

FAMILY AND SOCIAL ISSUES

Common reactions of parents who have a child with epilepsy include the development of feelings of guilt, anxiety and reactive depression. The desire of parents to do something compensatory for their impaired child and to concomitantly do something tangible to mitigate their own feelings of distress leads many parents to overprotect and/or overindulge the youngster with epilepsy. Similar considerations may complicate the efforts of teachers or others whose good intentions of helping the disadvantaged child with epilepsy may be subverted by their inadvertently presenting numerous opportunities for the youngster to exploit the illness for secondary gain.

The converse problem may also occur. Namely, parents used to expecting a given level of academic and social functioning from a child prior to the development of a seizure disorder may become inappropriately punitive and harsh in insisting that this level be maintained subsequently. Many parents and teachers are insufficiently aware of the cognitive and social impairments which a seizure disorder and anticonvulsant medication can generate. All these factors point to the need to involve parents and other caretakers in understanding and managing the psychiatric complications of epilepsy, including psychogenic seizures.

Comparably important to appreciate is the common experience of social rejection and ostracism by peers encountered by many epileptic youngsters. This reaction, often stemming from the fear and ignorance regarding epilepsy among the school-aged population, may accentuate the tendency of epileptic youngsters to utilize their illness as a way of getting compensatory attention from adults who often tend to be more supportive in this regard. As previously noted, the same mechanism may be utilized by a nonepileptic youngster who feels dejected or alienated for whatever reason and gleans indirectly or directly that special help and attention will be forthcoming if a "seizure" is produced.

DIFFERENTIAL DIAGNOSIS FOR PSYCHOTHERAPEUTIC/ PSYCHOBIOLOGICAL INTERVENTION

The clinical importance of determining the specific type of seizure disorder as a prerequisite for appropriate anticonvulsant drug treatment is well recognized. Differential diagnosis is also important in determining the possible merits of psychotherapeutic intervention with seizure patients. The most crucial distinction to make in this regard is between primary neurogenic seizures and those which are exclusively or primarily of psychological origin. It should be noted, however, that there are important subdivisions and tricky areas of possible overlap between these two major categories.

Psychogenic Precipitation of Neurogenic Seizures

The clinical literature on epilepsy contains many references to the role of environmental stress and emotional experiences as precipitants of seizures (Commission for the Control of Epilepsy and its Consequences, 1977; Minter, R., 1979). Several workers have reported emotional activation of the EEG in patients with convulsive disorders, particularly those with psychomotor and sensory epilepsy (Groethuysen et al., 1957; Stevens, 1962; Stevens and Milstein, 1964). Mignone et al. (1970) note that 53% of their 151 patients who had unequivocally abnormal EEGs reported precipitation of seizures by stress. Furthermore, the direct emotional activation of seizures has been documented with pentylenetetrazol-treated mice (Swinyard et al., 1963), genetically susceptible dogs (Martinek and Horak, 1970), and alumina cream epileptic rhesus monkeys (Kopeloff et al., 1954; Lockard et al., 1972) when these animals were exposed to various forms of environmental stress.

It therefore seems reasonable to posit that psychotherapy and related techniques that enable the patient and his or her family to deal more effectively with the emotional trauma of uncontrolled seizures, as well as with other environmental and intrapsychic stresses, could be helpful adjunctive aids in psychological and, hence, neurophysiological stabilization. This hypothesis is very difficult to substantiate empirically because of the methodological complexities involved. Nevertheless, cumulated clinical experience suggests that psychotherapeutic and related psychobiological techniques can sometimes contribute to breaking the cycle of repetitive, seizure-inducing psychophysiological activation that appears to occur in some patients whose seizures are not controlled by medication alone (Glaser, 1975; Mostofsky and Balaschak, 1977; Williams et al., 1979). With any type of neurogenic seizure disorder, therefore, it is important in the course of history taking and ongoing clinical assessment to determine, insofar as possible, to what extent emotional factors may play a role in precipitating the seizures.

Psychogenic Seizures

With the advent of the third edition of the Diagnostic and Statistical Manual of Mental Disorders (DSM-III), recently published by the American Psychiatric Association (Task Force on Nomenclature and Statistics of the American Psychiatric Association, 1980), seizures or seizure-like phenomena of primarily psychological origin are now most usefully subdivided into the following categories:

Factitious Seizures. Factitious disorders are characterized by physical or psychological symptoms that are produced by the patient and are under the patient's voluntary control. The judgment that a particular piece of behavior is under voluntary control is made by exclusion after all involuntary mechanisms for the behavior have been considered. When in doubt on this score, it is usually wiser to give the patient the benefit of this doubt and interpret to the youngster and family the plausibility of an unconscious mechanism. This face-saving maneuver will often be helpful in establishing a therapeutic alliance with the youngster as a means of facilitating symptom relinquishment. Only after persistent or repeated failure of this supportive approach would a more confrontational stance by the psychotherapist seem justified.

Somatoform Disorders. This term denotes a group of disorders that suggest organic illness for which there are no organic findings to explain the symptoms and for which there is positive evidence that the symptoms are linked to psychological factors. As with factitious illness and malingering, a somatoform disorder may coexist with a true neurogenic seizure disorder. Unlike factitious illness or malingering, the symptom production in somatoform disorders is not under voluntary control. That is, the patient does not have conscious awareness of controlling production or withdrawal of the symptoms.

Somatization Disorder (Briquet's Syndrome). This is a chronic but fluctuating disorder which begins early in life, often during childhood or adolescence, and is characterized by recurrent and multiple somatic complaints for which medical attention is sought but which are not apparently due to any physical illness. Complaints of at least 14 symptoms for females and 12 for males from the 37 listed in the DSM-III manual are required to establish the diagnosis (Task Force on Nomenclature and Statistics of the American Psychiatric Association, 1980). Anxiety and depressive features are common. In addition, abuse of alcohol and other drugs and diverse forms of antisocial behavior are frequently encountered. This syndrome is most common in adolescent girls and young women. It may include the presence of conversion seizures and is often associated with a histrionic personality disorder.

Conversion (Hysterical) Seizures. These symptoms have traditionally been explained as serving the purpose of reducing conflict-generated anxiety by keeping the conflict out of awareness while at the same time permitting it to be expressed symbolically. Conversion seizures usually develop in a setting of severe psychological stress such as experiencing intense conflict over sexual, aggressive or dependency needs. Yet the patient may display "la belle indifference," reflecting a relative lack of concern in view of the seriousness of the symptom. This feature of apparent calmness may be of dubious diagnostic value, however, since it is not always present with conversion seizures and it may be present in patients with neurogenic seizures who are stoical about their situation. There are often secondary gains evident on a careful review of the history with the patient and family. These may include avoiding noxious activities or getting support from the environment. In the clinical experience of the author, conversion seizures are the form of pseudoseizure most commonly encountered in children and adolescents.

Malingering. Here, seizures are consciously and voluntarily feigned. Moreover, this is done in pursuit of a goal which, when known, is obviously recognizable with an understanding of the individual's circumstances. Examples of this type of goal would include avoiding school, work, or military service, obtaining financial compensation, evading criminal prosecution, and obtaining drugs.

Intermittent Explosive Disorder (Rage Outbursts). This disorder is characterized by several discrete episodes of loss of control of aggressive impulses, resulting in serious assault or destruction of property. The behavior is grossly out of proportion to any precipitating psychosocial stressor and there is an absence of signs of generalized impulsivity or aggressiveness between episodes. In the experience of the author and others, this disorder is most often encountered in children and adolescents who have organic brain dysfunction, including epilepsy (Williams et al., 1979). Rage outbursts may also occur in association with conduct disorder in children and adolescents, often with associated organic brain dysfunction. As shall be noted later, rage outbursts may be specifically responsive to pharmacological intervention.

Characteristics of Psychogenic Seizures. The following characteristics may be delineated as favoring a diagnosis of "seizure-like phenomena" or pseudoseizures under the various categories outlined above, as distinct from true neurogenic seizures (Solomon and Plum, 1976):

1. The seizures emerge under stressful circumstances with an apparent primary gain of anxiety alleviation.
2. There are secondary gains, such as getting attention, being excused from school or work, collecting financial compensation, or escaping from an intolerable social situation.
3. There are other conversion symptoms and/or histrionic personality features.
4. The patient is hypnotizable and can recall the details of the seizure under hypnosis (Peterson et al., 1950; Schwarz et al., 1955; Sumner et al., 1952).
5. The seizures fail to conform to a physiologic pattern.
6. There is generally no incontinence during the attack, and, after the attack, one observes none of the drowsiness or depression of either stretch reflexes or oculovestibular (caloric) response that characterizes most epilepsy.
7. The tongue is rarely bitten, and the patient does not generally injure himself.

8. Corneal reflexes are present and plantar reflexes are flexor.
9. The EEG during the seizure is normal and shows no postictal slowing.

The more of the above criteria which are met, the greater the likelihood that a "seizure-like phenomenon" or pseudoseizure rather than a true neurogenic seizure has occurred. Further, it should be noted that some of these criteria are more discriminating than others, with EEG monitoring during the seizure being most specific if it can be obtained (Ramani et al., 1980).

Diagnostic Difficulties. It should be noted that even the experienced psychotherapist may encounter difficulty in ascertaining the level of the patient's awareness of relevant psychodynamic issues leading to a pseudoseizure (Williams et al., 1979).

Additionally, it may be impossible for the clinician, even when observing a given seizure, to be certain about the distinction between a pseudoseizure and a psychogenically precipitated neurogenic seizure, unless there is the benefit of ongoing EEG monitoring. This is especially true when a psychomotor (partial complex) seizure is in question, because the presentation may be so atypical (Remick and Wada, 1979).

Finally, just as any of the various subtypes of psychogenic seizures may occur in a patient with a coexisting neurogenic seizure disorder, so also different forms of psychogenic seizures may occur in the same patient over time. The above categories may, therefore, be most usefully thought of as part of a spectrum of possible but not necessarily mutually exclusive psychopathological determinants of seizures. Often, ongoing assessment of the patient and family over a period of time is needed to clarify these issues. Furthermore, sometimes even after successful symptom control, the diagnostic question may not be fully resolved.

OVERVIEW OF PSYCHOTHERAPEUTIC/ PSYCHOBIOLOGICAL TREATMENT STRATEGIES

A broad spectrum of techniques that are part of the general armamentarium of both dynamically and behaviorally trained practitioners have been applied to the control of seizure disorders (Mostofsky and Balaschak, 1977). It is, however, extremely difficult, if not impossible, to examine any one psychotherapeutic procedure independent of other overlapping or concurrent therapeutic influences. In part this is because the environmental and intrapsychic triggers of seizures are often complex and multidetermined, so that treatment programs are commonly designed to attack more than a single objective. In fact, almost all studies cited below implicitly or explicitly combine more than a single category of procedure in a given therapy program.

The treatment and strategies below have been grouped under the headings of Conditioning Techniques, Psychodynamic Approaches, Relaxation and Hypnosis, Biofeedback and Pharmacological Interventions. Reports are cited to illustrate the diversity of approaches that have been reported to be successfully applied in the treatment of seizure disorders. Each of the references cited describes either one or a few cases in which the particular strategy applied led to improved seizure control as compared to pretreatment baseline frequency. It should be noted that reports describing both neurogenic and psychogenic seizures are included, as are cases involving children, adolescents and adults. Individual reports are not always rigorous in distinguishing between neurogenic and psychogenic seizures nor in controlling for possible effects of unreported medication changes. With the exception of habituation training in various forms of sensory-evoked epilepsies and propranolol for rage outbursts, no effort is made in the list of treatment approaches below to establish specificity of treatment and correlate this with the diagnostic categories outlined above. The field is at too early a stage of development for these types of connections to be generally established with conviction. It is hoped, however, that greater precision in differential diagnosis and in systematic study of treatment interventions will allow greater clarity regarding specificity and efficacy of treatment to emerge in the course of further research.

Conditioning Techniques

Conditioning techniques include denial of reward, penalty program, relief (avoidance), punishment, overt and covert rewards and habituation (extinction).

Denial of Reward. Attentive concern toward the patient may tend to positively reinforce seizures. Thus the reward denial paradigm requires that the occurrence of a seizure is not followed by a display of care, concern, or indeed any attention. The seizure is ignored, as one might ignore some other undesirable behavior such as a tantrum. The expectation is that continued nonrecognition of this behavior will lead to its extinction (Gardner, 1967).

Penalty Program. In this procedure, when the patient has a seizure he or she is asked to enter a "time-out room" or equivalent environment in which he or she does not have access to reinforcement. As contrasted to the "denial of reward" category, rather than passive ignoring of the behavior this approach required that the observer intervene and react to the patient. In an institutional setting, this may involve moving a patient from an open ward to a less open setting or denying the patient visits or off-ground privileges. In a home or school setting with a child, this might entail denying the child a recess period or another favorite activity. It is explained to the patient that such action is being taken so that he or she will no longer be in danger, and it is explained that he or she will be able to return to previous activities when his or her condition improves (Richardson, 1972).

Relief Avoidance Program. In this procedure an aversive stimulus, such as photic stimulation during a spike-and-wave paroxysm appearing on an EEG record, is administered. Administration of the noxious agent is continued until the subject demonstrates a reduction in either the clinical or the electrical manifestations of the seizures (Ounsted et al., 1966).

Punishment Program. In this program, a seizure is immediately followed by the administration of a noxious stimulus, such as an annoying electric shock, or a noise, or a flash of light (Efron, 1956 and 1957; Wright, 1973).

Overt Reward Program. In this technique, following totally seizure-free periods of time or following a particular time period during which there is a significant decrease in seizure rate, rewards are administered. The criterion of a seizure-free time is gradually extended or the allowable number of seizures per unit time is gradually reduced in an attempt to achieve full seizure control (Zlutnick et al., 1975).

Covert Reward Program. Seizure-provoking and non-seizure-provoking scenes are suggested to the patient while he or she is in a relaxed state. These scenes are immediately followed by imagined scenes of appropriate reward or nonreward as indicated. No tangible token, privilege, praise or punishment is given; only the imagined representation is suggested to the patient (Daniels, 1975).

Habituation or Extinction. Forster (1972), using classical conditioning techniques, has done much work in habituation training of various stimulus-evoked epilepsies. Where seizures are sensorially precipitated, this treatment strategy stipulates that the stimulus be presented below threshold and the intensity or frequency be gradually increased until the stimulus loses its seizure-evocative capacity.

Comment. With the exception of Forster's work on habituation, frequently conducted with adult outpatients, conditioning strategies in the forms outlined above are most readily applied with children, with retarded patients and with those in institutional settings. In these instances the therapist has greater potential control over the contingencies of positive or negative reinforcement than with the more autonomously functioning adolescent. In the latter case, the same principles of reward management may be applicable, but they may be operationally more effective if integrated with a strategy for self-control, such as psychotherapy. In most instances, it requires a patient with greater ego strengths to successfully negotiate a strategy predicated on self-mastery.

Psychodynamic Approaches

Psychodynamic approaches include psychotherapy and the identification of emotional triggers.

Psychoanalytically Oriented Psychotherapy. Gottschalk (1953) describes how the seizure frequencies of three epileptic children, each with EEG documentation of diagnosis and each of whose seizures were not controlled by medication, decreased notably during and after a course of dynamically oriented psychotherapy consisting of at least one hundred individual sessions. The author cites evidence that both interpersonal events as well as intrapersonal conflicts activated epileptic behavior in these children. Elsewhere (Gottschalk, 1956), he elaborates further on his thesis of the value of psychoanalytic psychotherapy in the management of certain types of epileptic patients.

Identifying Emotional Triggers. Feldman and Paul (1976) describe a technique of simulated recall and video replay which reduced seizure frequency in 5 patients with psychomotor epilepsy, documented by EEG and not controlled by medication. The authors contend that previous psychotherapeutic efforts had been unsuccessful antecedent message-input which had triggered the seizures. Using video taping of seizures and antecedent triggering events seemed helpful in enabling patients to either avoid or better cope with threatening environmental events.

Comment. The role of psychoanalytically oriented psychotherapy in the treatment of somatoform disorders and, hence, conversion seizures is generally accepted (Nemiah, 1980). What is not clear is why psychotherapy should be effective in the management of psychogenically precipitated neurogenic seizures. One plausible hypothesis may draw upon the frequently found suppression or limitation of paroxysmal activity during states of attention, stimulation, and concentration, particularly during periods of interest and high motivation (Glaser, 1975). A related postulate in this hypothesis is that these qualities of altered central nervous system arousal are part of the essential ingredients of any successful psychotherapeutic strategy and are indeed sustained in the patient if the psychotherapy is successful (Frank et al., 1978). This theoretical frame of reference remains to be substantiated by further research.

Relaxation and Hypnosis

Relaxation techniques include relaxation, desensitization, and hypnosis.

Relaxation. All of the relaxation therapies share the features of muscular relaxation, regular practice, mental focusing, and task awareness (Cabral and Scott, 1976; Mostofsky and Vicks, 1973).

Desensitization. In this approach, the patient is instructed to systematically relax and then think of a progressive hierarchy of anxiety-provoking scenes which had previously been established, by observation of the patient, to be seizure-provoking (Parrino, 1971).

Hypnosis. The role of hypnosis as an adjunctive aid in various somatoform disorders, including conversion seizures, is well documented (Spiegel and Spiegel, 1978; Williams and Singh, 1976). Additional reports (Gardner, 1967; Stein, 1963; Williams et al. 1978) suggest that the stabilizing effects of hypnosis may also be of value in psychogenically triggered neurogenic seizures.

Comment. Reasoning by analogy may well be justified in this realm for heuristic purposes. Controlled studies of various relaxation therapies have shown each of them to be superior to placebo and some to be superior to other techniques in treating certain psychophysiologic disorders. For example, in a review of various forms of relaxation therapy used as adjunctive aids in the clinical management of hypertension. Jacob et al. (1977) found that superior and more sustained results were achieved by strategies employing various forms of relaxation therapy as compared with those strategies employing only formal biofeedback procedures. Whether similar findings will be documented in the area of seizure disorders remains to be clarified by further research. Clinical experience suggests that for seizure patients relaxation techniques should be used in combination with other methods, such as supportive psychotherapy or biofeedback.

Biofeedback

Biofeedback entails operant conditioning. The patient is instructed to generate or avoid generating a given bioelectric pattern or waveform during ongoing EEG monitoring. Correct or incorrect responses are appropriately fed back (for example, by visual or auditory signal) and may be actively rewarded or punished. The detailed and experimentally rigorous work of Sterman and co-workers (1973, 1974, 1978), Wyler and co-workers (1976, 1979) and Kuhlman (1978) cannot be adequately addressed here. The implications of their work, however, may be summarized as follows (Kuhlman, 1978):

1. Significant seizure reductions can occur with EEG feedback training which are not related to placebo effects, nonspecific factors or to changes in medication.
2. EEG changes associated with such training can best be described as "normalization."
3. Continued clinical investigation of EEG feedback training as a nonpharmacological adjunct to conventional therapy appears justified.

PHARMACOLOGICAL INTERVENTIONS

A recent report (Williams et al., 1982) suggests that propranolol, a β-adrenergic blocking agent, may have specific benefits in treating children and adolescents who have uncontrolled rage outbursts associated with organic brain dysfunction. In this report of 30 patients, 14 had a documented diagnosis of neurogenic seizures independent of their rage outbursts. All patients had prior unsuccessful treatment with medication, including analeptics, neuroleptics, anticonvulsants, or combinations of these. The majority of the sample also had prior psychotherapeutic intervention, all without success. In this retrospective study, more than 75% of the patients, all of whom received propranolol, had moderate to marked improvement in control of rage outbursts and aggressive behavior. A controlled prospective study is suggested to substantiate these findings.

In the author's experience, some youngsters with pseudoseizures as well as some with psychogenically precipitated neurogenic seizures have benefited from gradually augmented doses of imipramine when depression was clinically evident. Caution is warranted here, however. Although imipramine has been demonstrated to have anticonvulsant effects in some patients with absence and myoclonic-astatic seizures (Fromm et al., 1978), it has also been reported to induce or exacerbate grand mal and partial complex seizures in some patients at higher doses (Lange et al., 1976).

The use of neuroleptics in children and adolescents having psychogenic seizures should be restricted to those with documented diagnoses of pervasive developmental disorders or acute psychotic episodes. This is primarily because of the tendency of neuroleptics to lower the seizure threshold and also because of the lack of substantial benefit from neuroleptics for other diagnostic categories in children and adolescents. Although diazepam could safely be used if an anxiolytic were needed, the author has rarely found it to be of benefit in youngsters with psychogenic seizures because of its tendency to cause sedation and exacerbate depression.

DISCUSSION OF SPECIALIZED TREATMENT TECHNIQUES

The preceding discussion of treatment techniques indicates the multiplicity of approaches that have been used as adjuncts in the management of uncontrolled seizures and their many variants. These numerous techniques are not mutually exclusive; in fact, they are often combined in practice. They may, indeed, share common features—such as progressive relaxation, attention activation, generation of positive expectancies, implicit or explicit reward/punishment features, and emotional support—that are more uniformly operative in each than the proponents of the different methodologies might readily acknowledge. As a group, the reports of these treatments call attention to the interaction of environmental, interpersonal, intrapsychic and neurophysiologic factors in influencing the frequency of seizures and pseudoseizures in many patients. Indeed, in some of the reports cited, not only was improved seizure control achieved by the stated intervention but also this improvement was maintained to a degree allowing substantial reduction of anticonvulsant doses, with consequent diminution of associated side effects.

Of the treatment techniques discussed, the recent studies in EEG feedback training have the advantage of most methodological precision, controlled experimental design, and hence greatest demonstrated specificity in ruling out placebo effects. However, these advantages are somewhat offset at present by the rather elaborate and expensive technology required for effective EEG feedback training and monitoring, which limits its availability. If the favorable results of some workers in this area continue to be sustained by further studies, it seems probable that advances in miniaturization and mass production of training and monitoring components could readily enhance their availability.

An alternate or complementary consideration might entail exploring the psychological correlates of EEG "normalization." This could involve EEG-monitored studies of the purported process of "normalized" central nervous system arousal, which has been posited as the mechanism of efficacy of the conditioning, psychotherapy and relaxation strategies previously outlined. From another perspective, it could involve careful psychometric assessment of the emotional and cognitive correlates of EEG feedback training, which has not been done in detail to date. It is of interest that Cobb (1940), using eclectically based psychiatric treatment of carefully selected drug-resistant seizure patients in the days antedating biofeedback availability, obtained results similar to those of the best current biofeedback workers, in terms of percentage of favorable clinical responders (67% showed marked improvement and 10% showed slight improvement).

The recent report of propranolol in the treatment of paroxysmal rage outbursts in children and adolescents (Williams et al., 1982) highlights the fact that pharmacological approaches beyond the existing regimen of anticonvulsant medication clearly merit consideration in the treatment of seizure-like phenomena.

Perhaps the most important therapeutic generalizations to emphasize for psychologists and psychiatrists treating children and adolescents with psychogenic seizures are the need to individualize their care and the need to involve the parents as well as significant others in the treatment as productively as possible. Parents usually constitute the most potent influenceable variable in the child's or adolescent's environment. Most of the above outlined interventions require their consent and work more effectively if the patient perceives his parents' consensual validation and the neurologist's support for their use. Maintaining a simultaneous trusting and cooperative rapport with the patient, parents and treating neurologist, therefore, seems to be one of the prerequisites for success in the treatment of children and adolescents with psychogenic seizures.

Just as no single anticonvulsant medication has emerged that is uniformly efficacious for all neurogenic seizure patients, so also is no single psychotherapeutic or psychobiological modality uniformly effective in all cases of pseudoseizures or psychogenically precipitated neurogenic seizures (Williams et al., 1979). As the neurologist may need to go through multiple clinical trials in attempting to formulate an anticonvulsant regimen best suited to a patient's need, so must the mental health practitioner be prepared to reformulate his or her treatment strategy based on the patient's pattern of response. It follows logically that it behooves the practitioner to have a diversified therapeutic armamentarium available to this end.

References

Cabral, R. J., and Scott, D. S. The effects of desensitization techniques, biofeedback, and relaxation on intractable epilepsy: Follow-up study. *J. Neurol. Neurosurg. Psychiatry* 39:504–507, 1976.

Cantwell, D.P. Hyperkinetic syndrome. In *Child Psychiatry: Modern Approaches*, edited by Rutter, M., and Hersov, L. Blackwell, London, 1977, pp. 524–555.

Cobb, S. Psychiatric approach to the treatment of epilepsy. *Am. J. Psychiatry* 96:1009, 1940.

Commission for the Control of Epilepsy and its Consequences. *Plan for Nationwide Action on Epilepsy.* U.S. Dept. of H.E.W., National Institutes of Health, Bethesda, 1977, part 2, pp. 393–402.

Daniels, L. The treatment of grand mal epilepsy by covert and operant conditioning techniques: A case study. *Psychosom. Med. 16*:65–67, 1975.

Desai, B. T., Riley, T. L., Porter, R. J., et al. Active noncompliance as a cause of uncontrolled seizures. *Epilepsia 19*:447–452, 1978.

Efron, R. The effect of olfactory stimuli in arresting uncinate fits. *Brain 79*:267–281, 1956.

Efron, R. The conditioned inhibition of uncinate fits. *Brain 80*:251–252, 1957.

Feldman, R., and Paul, N. Identity of emotional triggers in epilepsy. *J. Nerv. Ment. Dis. 162*:345–353, 1976.

Forster, F. The classification and condition of the reflex epilepsies. *Int. J. Neurol. 9*:73–86, 1972.

Frank, J.D., Hoehn-Saric, Imber, S.D., et al. *Effective Ingredients of Successful Psychotherapy.* Brunner/Mazel, New York, 1978.

Fromm, G., Wessel, H. Glass, J., et al. Imipramine in absence and myoclonic-astatic seizures. *Neurology 28*:953–957, 1978.

Gardner, G. Use of hypnosis for psychogenic epilepsy in a child. *Am. J. Clin. Hypn. 15*: 166–169, 1973.

Gardner, J. Behavior therapy treatment approach to a psychogenic seizure case. *J. Consult. Psychol. 31*:209–212, 1967.

Glaser, G. Epilepsy-neuropsychological aspects. In *American Handbook of Psychiatry*, vol. IV, edited by Reiser, M. Basic Books, New York, 1975, pp. 314–355.

Glaser, G. Convulsive disorders. In *Textbook of Neurology*, ed. 6, edited by Merritt, H.H. Lea & Febiger, Philadelphia, 1979, pp. 843–882.

Gottschalk, L. Effects of intensive psychotherapy on epileptic children. *Arch. Neurol. Psychiatry 70*:361–384, 1953.

Gottschalk, L. The relationship of psychologic state and epileptic child. In *The Psychoanalytic Study of the Child.* Yale University Press, New Haven, 1956.

Groethuysen, U.C., Robinson, D.B., Haylett, C.H., et al. Depth electrogenic recording of a seizure during a structured interview. *Psychosom. Med. 19*:353–362, 1957.

Jacob, R.G., Kraemer, H.C., and Agras, W.S. Relaxation therapy in the treatment of hypertension. *Arch. Gen. Psychiatry 34*:1417–1427, 1977.

Kopeloff, L.M., Chusid, J.G., and Kopeloff, N. Chronic experimental epilepsy in Macaca mulatta. *Neurology 4*:218–227, 1954.

Kuhlman, W.N. EEG feedback training of epileptic patients: Clinical and electroencephalographic analysis. *Electroencehpalogr. Clin. Neurophysiol. 45*:699–710, 1978.

Lange, S.C., Julien, R.M., and Fowler, G.W. Biphasic effects of imipramine in experimental models of epilepsy. *Epilepsia 17*:183–196, 1976.

Lockard, J.S., Wilson, W.L., and Uhlir, V. Spontaneous seizure frequency and avoidance conditioning in monkeys. *Epilepsia 13*:437–444, 1972.

Martinek, Z., and Horak, F. Development of so-called genuine epileptic seizures in dogs during emotional excitement. *Physiol. Bohemoslov. 19*:185–195, 1970.

Mignone, R.J., Donnelly, E.F., and Sadowsky, O. Psychological and neurological comparisons of psychomotor and nonpsychomotor epileptic patients. *Epilepsia 11*:345, 1970.

Minter, R.E. Can emotions precipitate seizures: A review of the question. *J. Fam. Pract. 8*: 55–59, 1979.

Mostofsky, D.I., and Balaschak, B. Psychobiological control of seizures. *Psychol. Bull. 84*: 723–750, 1977.

Mostofsky, D.I., and Vicks, S.H. The therapeutic value of muscle relaxation in seizure control: A case study. unpublished manuscript, 1973.

Nemiah, J.C. Somatoform disorders. In *Comprehensive Textbook of Psychiatry*, ed. 3, edited by Kaplan, H., Freedman, A., and Sadock, B. Williams & Wilkins, Baltimore, 1980, pp. 1483–1492.

Ounsted, C., Lee, D., and Hutt, S.J. Electroencephalographic and clinical changes in an epileptic child during repeated photic stimulation. *Electroencephalogr. Clin. Neurophysiol. 21*:388–391, 1966.

Parrino, J. Reduction of seizures by desensitization. *J. Behav. Ther. Exp. Psychiatry 2*:215–218, 1971.

Peterson, D.B., Sumner, J.N., and Jones, G.A. Role of hypnosis in differentiation of epileptic from convulsive-like seizures. *Am. J. Psychiatry 107*:428–432, 1950.

Ramani, S.V., Quesney, F.F., Olson, D., et al. Diagnosis of hysterical seizures in epileptic patients. *Am. J. Psychiatry* 137:705–709, 1980.

Remick, R.A., and Wada, J.A. Complex partial and pseudoseizure disorders. *Am. J. Psychiatry* 136:320–323, 1979.

Richardson, R. Environmental contingencies in seizure disorders. Presented at the Association for Advancement of Behavioral Therapy, New York, 1972.

Schwarz, B.E., Bickford, R.G., and Rasmussen, W.C. Hypnotic phenomena, including hypnotically activated seizures, studies with the EEG. *J. Nerv. Ment. Dis.* 122:564–574, 1955.

Shaffer, D. Brain injury. In *Child Psychiatry: Modern Approaches*, edited by Rutter, M. and Hersov, L. Blackwell, London, 1977, pp. 185–215.

Solomon, G., and Plum, F. *Clinical Management of Seizures*. Saunders, Philadelphia, 1976.

Spiegel, H., and Spiegel, D. *Trance and Treatment: Clinical Uses of Hypnosis*. Basic Books, New York, 1978.

Stein, C. The clenched fist technique as a hypnotic procedure in clinical psychotherapy. *Am. J. Clin. Hypn.* 6:113–119, 1963.

Sterman, M. Neurophysiologic and clinical studies of sensorimotor EEG biofeedback training: Some effects on epilepsy. *Semin. Psychiatry* 5:507–525, 1973.

Sterman, M., et al. Biofeedback training of the sensorimotor EEG rhythm in man: Effects on epilepsy. *Epilepsia* 15:395–416, 1974.

Sterman, M., and Macdonald, L.T. Effects of central cortical EEG feedback training on incidence of poorly controlled seizures. *Epilepsia* 19:207–222, 1978.

Stevens, J.R. Central and peripheral factors in epileptic discharge. *Arch. Neurol.* 7:330–338, 1962.

Stevens, J.R., and Milstein, V. Electroclinical correlates of emotional activation of the electroencephalogram. *J. Nerv. Ment. Dis.* 138:146–155, 1964.

Sumner, J.W., Rameron, R.R., and Peterson, D.B. Hypnosis in differentiation of epileptic from convulsive-like seizures. *Neurology* 2:395–402, 1952.

Swinyard, E.A., Miyahara, J.T., Clark, L.D., et al. The effect of experimentally induced stress on pentylenetetrazol threshold in mice. *Psychopharmacologia* 4:343–353, 1963.

Task Force on Nomenclature and Statistics of the American Psychiatric Association. *Diagnostic and Statistical Manual of Mental Disorders*, ed. 3. American Psychiatric Association, New York, 1980.

Williams, D.T., Gold, A.P., Shrout, P., et al. The impact of psychiatric intervention on patients with uncontrolled seizures. *J. Nerv. Ment. Dis.* 167:626–631, 1979.

Williams, D.T., Mehl, R., Yudofsky, S.C., et al. The effect of propranolol on uncontrolled rage outbursts in children and adolescents with organic brain dysfunction. *J. Am. Acad. Child. Psychiatry*, 1982, in press.

Williams, D.T., and Singh, M. Hypnosis as a facilitating therapeutic adjunct in child psychiatry. *J. Am. Acad. Child Psychiatry* 15:326–342, 1976.

Williams, D.T., Spiegel, H., and Mostofsky, D.I. Neurogenic and hysterical seizures in children and adolescents: Differential diagnostic and therapeutic considerations. *Am. J. Psychiatry* 135:82–86, 1978.

Wright, L. Aversive conditioning of self-induced seizures. *Behav. Res. Ther.* 4:712–713, 1973.

Wyler, A.R., Lockard, J.S., Ward, A.A., et al. Conditioned EEG desychronization and seizure occurrence in patients. *Electroencephalogr. Clin. Neurophysiol.* 41:501–512, 1976.

Wyler, A.R., Robbins, C.A., and Dodrill, C.B. EEG operant conditioning for control of epilepsy. *Epilepsia* 20:279–286, 1979.

Zlutnick, S, et al. Behavioral control of seizure disorders. In *Behavior Therapy and Health Care: Principles and Applications*, edited by Katz, R., and Zlutnick, S. Pergamon Press, New York, 1975.

 # Aggression and Epilepsy

ERNST A. RODIN, M.D.

To a superficial observer, it might seem inappropriate to include a chapter of this type in a book which deals with "Pseudoseizures," but, as will be shown, the overwhelming majority of serious criminal acts attributed to epilepsy occur in individuals who have a history of "spells" or "seizures" which do not fit into any of the currently recognized forms of epilepsy.

In order to do some justice to this exceedingly complex field, the following outline will be employed:

1. A discussion of how violence or aggression has become linked to epilepsy, with a review of the clinical literature.
2. A review of the electroencephalographic literature, which will include interictal, ictal, and depth electrographic results.
3. A review of individual case reports from the literature.
4. A review of the literature placing the problem in numerical perspective.
5. Information developed at a recent workshop sponsored by the Epilepsy Foundation of America on the topic of Epilepsy and Violent/Aggressive Behavior.
6. Personal experiences of this author, including a case report.
7. Theoretical formulation of possible neurophysiologic mechanisms, with suggestions for future research.
8. The legal dilemma and guidelines for medicolegal testimony.

THE SHAPING OF MODERN IDEAS ON EPILEPSY AND AGGRESSIVE BEHAVIOR

The earliest recorded instance of connecting epilepsy with violent behavior is recorded by Herodotus in the discussion of the behavior of Cambyses, King of Persia, who reigned between 529 and 522 B.C. Among his numerous impulsive acts the one of killing the son of a trusted servant in a fit of anger, who happened to be an innocent bystander during one of the King's arguments, is most relevant in this context. What is important is that the King's epilepsy was of early onset and was accompanied by a violent, irascible temperament associated with abuse of alcohol. Had he not been a king, but a commoner, and had he shot the son of one of his friends with a gun in the 1970s, it is extremely likely that epilepsy would have been used as a legal defense as it was during the trial of Jack Ruby. The history related in both instances indicates clearly, however, that the crimes were purposeful, the individuals had complete recall, and their actions could therefore not have been a direct result of an epileptic seizure.

It was known from early times that epileptic individuals may have associated serious mental problems. The first statistical data on the incidence of mental disturbances among epileptic patients was presented by Esquirol (Temkin, 1971). Since the figures were derived from an institutionalized group, they are obviously biased toward mental pathology but need to be cited for background information. Eighty percent of 399 epileptic women were regarded as "mentally affected." Of these, 38% had dementia, 12% had periodic memory loss, 10% had mania, and 8.5% had "fury." The rest showed a variety of characterologic difficulties. The terms "epileptic mania" and "epileptic fury," which later became "furor epilepticus" and "raving fits," are important because from them derived the notion that in these "epileptic" attacks the patient might commit murder. By the late eighteenth and early nineteenth century, the definition of epilepsy, which in earlier times was of course limited to the "falling sickness," became broadened and the concept of "mania transitoria" emerged, namely, passing states of maniacal excitement which occur as substitutes for the more typical epileptic attacks. During the nineteenth century, these ideas became generally accepted and they are still exerting their influence in the last quarter of the twentieth century. In 1874 Maudsley wrote

> Certainly the most desperate instances of homicidal impulses are met in conjunction with epilepsy. The homicidal mania may take the place of the ordinary epileptic convulsion being truly a masked epilepsy. The diseased action has been transferred from one nervous center to another and instead of a convulsion of muscles, the patient is seized with a convulsion of ideas.

Lest one believe that the term "masked epilepsy" has been discarded, it should be mentioned that Tippett and Pine presented case examples in 1957 under the same title.

The difference in opinions on this topic and the basic split between neurologic and psychiatric views are evident in the concise writings of

Hughlings-Jackson, who around 1870 took issue with the concept of "masked epilepsy" and laid the foundations of our current ideas as to what is and what is not epilepsy (Jackson and Taylor, 1958). It is impossible to do justice to Hughling-Jackson's writings in this chapter and the reader is therefore most strongly urged to consult the original, especially the paper entitled "On Temporary Mental Disorders after Epileptic Paroxysms" (1958). In brief, Jackson held that the essential element of epilepsy is "the paroxysmal affection of consciousness." In order to have a term for the complex actions occurring after a seizure of which the individual is unaware and therefore cannot be held legally responsible, he used the words "mental automatism." He felt that automatic behavior always occurred as a postictal rather than an ictal event, even in those cases in which there was no apparent clinical seizure. "I believe there is in such cases during the paroxysm an internal discharge too slight to cause obvious external effect but strong enough to put out of use for a time more or less of the highest nervous centers." It is truly remarkable that this view is now fully supported by the evidence not only of scalp but even more so of depth electrography, as will be shown later in the appropriate context. In his case presentations he repeatedly made the point that "automatisms" are usually innocent, confused actions but could, under accidental circumstances, lead to dangerous and criminal conduct. The word "could" is important because his personal, extensive experience did not include a single case of directed, aggravated assault upon another person.

Turner, likewise a neurologist, used the term "psychical epilepsy" for

> incomplete acts frequently succeeded by a somnambulistic state or stage of automatism.... Sometimes there is violence, the patient striking or injuring those about him. On the other hand, he may carry out certain purposeful movements such as taking off his clothes or emptying his pockets.... It is not usual to find violence and assault ...; but there were two cases in which this was noted; in both, the assault was of a homicidal character; but *neither* patient was a genuine epileptic.

In agreement with Jackson, he took issue with the opinion that there are "psychical equivalents" for epilepsy: "It may indeed be categorically stated that there is no psychical equivalent condition, which is not also seen as a pre- or postconclusive phenomenon" (Turner, 1973).

Gowers, Jackson, and Turner seemed to have the largest personal experience with epileptic patients at that time and they had never seen a personal case of goal-directed murder as the result of an epileptic attack. The significance of their contemporary views can only be appreciated fully when one reads the views of Lombroso as expressed in

L'Uomo Delinquente. Lombroso's intent was to bring medical science to bear on the study of criminal behavior and to provide for a more humane penal system. The tragedy of his life was that the scientific methodology available to him could not provide the desired results. Also, his thesis was expressed in a manner that has done a great deal of harm to his overall cause and has lent an even greater stigma to individual patients with epilepsy. We have not yet recovered from the impact of his writings and they prevent, even today, the medical scientific studies of criminal behavior which are so urgently needed. "From Phrenology to Psychosurgery and Back Again: Biological Studies of Criminality" by Nassi and Abramowitz (1975) is a case in point. The following excerpts from Lombroso's work are taken from the book *Criminal Man According to the Classification of Cesare Lombroso* (Lombroso-Ferrero, 1972). In the most relevant chapter, entitled "Epileptics, and Their Relation to Born Criminals and the Morally Insane," Lombroso concludes:

> We have already stated that the physical and psychic characteristics of born criminals coincide with those of the morally insane. Both are identical with those of another class of degenerates, known to the world as epileptics. . . . Careful examination of epileptics by clinical and mental experts, showed that in addition to the characteristic seizures, these unfortunate beings were subject to other phenomena, which sometimes took the place of the convulsive fit and in other cases preceded or followed it. These were pavor nocturnus, sudden sweats, heat, neuralgia, sialorrhea, periodical cephalalgia and, above all, vertigo; and these symptoms were not always accompanied by unconsciousness nor followed by coma. Sometimes the seizure was only manifested by paroxysms of rage or ferocious and brutal impulses (devouring animals alive), which, if consciously committed, would be considered criminal. This fact led doctors and mental experts to examine other patients, and they were able to advance positive proof that a certain number of epileptics never experience the typical seizure, the disease being manifested in this milder form with cephalalgia, sialorrhea, delirious ferocity, and above all, giddiness.

This position is reiterated in the chapter on "The Insane Criminal"; under the subheading "Epilepsy," one finds:

> We have spoken of this disease in another chapter and have shown that the born criminal is in reality an epileptic, in whom the malady, instead of manifesting itself suddenly in strange muscular contortions or terrible spasms, develops slowly in continual brain irritation, which causes the individual thus affected to reproduce the ferocious egotism natural to primitive savages, irresistibly bent on harming others.

There is no point in belaboring the literature between the turn of the century and the middle of the 1950s because we find only variants of the same views. In critically assessing the literature as presented up to now, it is evident that there are basically two schools of thought: Epileptic patients could, but as a rule do not, injure someone as part of the ictal or postictal state, and any bodily harm that may be done by the patient in the interictal state is either a result of associated personality difficulties or concomitant psychosis of the interictal or postictal variety. The other school holds that the classical forms of epilepsy, as recognized by neurologists today, do not encompass the entire spectrum of epileptic manifestations and there exists a certain patient population which does not have recognized or recognizable epileptic seizures but suffers from "equivalents" which may take the form of autonomic symptoms, headaches, behavior disorders, or even criminal acts. This basic position of Falret, Maudsley, and Lombroso might have been discarded for lack of substantive evidence, but it keeps reappearing as a result of the use, as well as abuse, of electroencephalography.

THE ROLE OF ELECTROENCEPHALOGRAPHY IN THE ASSESSMENT OF VIOLENT BEHAVIOR

Berger's original hope that electroencephalography would allow discovery of the neural basis of mental functions has turned out to be illusory. It was natural, however, that mentally ill patients were extensively investigated. While a larger percentage of psychiatric patients were found to have EEG abnormalities than a comparable normal control population, no specific patterns emerged that would allow an unequivocal statement that a given person suffers from a specified psychiatric condition. It was noted quite early that among the various psychiatric patient populations, the group of "psychopaths" had the largest incidence of borderline or abnormal EEGs which consisted either of diffuse background slowing or paroxysmal activity with or without spike components (Hill and Watterston, 1942; Silverman, 1943). Stafford-Clark and Taylor (1949), who examined prisoners charged with murder, found that the highest rate of EEG abnormalities, 74%, occurred in individuals whose crimes were apparently motiveless or had minimal motive. The lowest rate, 10%, was found when murder was incidental to the commission of another crime. This entire study involved only 64 prisoners and has never been replicated in this manner, but it certainly deserves to be repeated.

Leaving aside erroneous overinterpretation of EEG data, one is left with a residue of patients who do not have clinical epilepsy but do show at times "epileptiform activity." The 6 cycle-per-second (cps) spike wave pattern as opposed to the 3 cps spike wave pattern of petit mal absence is, according to Hughes et al. (1965), more commonly associated with psychiatric problems, especially nervousness, depression, and emotional instability, than with overt seizures, and so is the 14 and 6 cps positive spike wave pattern as well as the psychomotor variant pattern. The 14 and 6 cps positive spike pattern is especially important in this context because it was originally described under the name of "thalamic and hypothalamic epilepsy" and there exist isolated case reports of adolescents with this pattern who have committed murder (Schwade and Geiger, 1953; Winfield and Ozturk, 1959). Inasmuch as the pattern is quite common in adolescents (20%) and murder is rather infrequent, a link between the two is extremely tenuous (Gibbs and Gibbs, 1963). The same applies to the psychomotor variant pattern which was supposedly present in Jack Ruby's electroencephalogram but, according to Gibbs and Gibbs who described this EEG finding (1952, 1963), it is mostly accompanied by dizziness, headache, nausea, and vomiting, as well as mild behavior disorders. Reviewing the symptoms described by Gibbs and Gibbs in the *Atlas of Electroencephalography* (1952) and said to accompany the "14 and 6" and the "psychomotor variant" patterns, one finds a remarkable resemblance (apart from the devouring of animals) to those that were listed by Lombroso as taking "the place of the convulsive fit." Gibbs and Gibbs stated in 1963: ". . . we believe that the weight of present evidence suggests that the classical types of epilepsy, which are recognizable and fairly accurately diagnosable from clinical symptomatology, do not include all the forms which epilepsy takes in man." Regardless of whether or not one believes that these patterns are epileptic, the fact remains that while 19% of patients with 14 and 6 cps positive spikes have rage reactions this has to be put into perspective by citing the study of Riley and Niedermeyer (1978) who examined 229 EEGs of 121 patients referred for episodic acts of violence unaccompanied by other neurologic disorders or psychosis and found only 6.6% to have been either minimally or slightly abnormal. None were found markedly abnormal and the percentage of abnormal records did not differ significantly from the incidence of abnormalities in the healthy population. It must also be mentioned that neither Gibbs and Gibbs *nor anyone else* has ever recorded the 14 and 6 cps positive spike or psychomotor variant pattern as part of a clinical seizure. Nevertheless, Gibbs and Gibbs (1963) felt that "Masked forms of epilepsy, however, are not clinically diagnosable and the borderland of epilepsy is an impassable morass without electroencephalographic guidance."

We are, therefore, left with the observation that patients with epileptic-like EEG manifestations exist who are either clinically asymptomatic or have a variety of episodic disturbances which are not clearly epileptic in nature and who may or may not respond to anticonvulsant medications. If we accept Hughlings-Jackson's definition of epilepsy being "a sudden, excessive neuronal discharge," then these episodic states would not qualify because the EEG as recorded from the scalp is always unchanged during these behavioral alterations. For a patient to have a given symptom definitely diagnosed as indeed epileptic in nature, one will have to insist that it is accompanied by recognizable seizure discharges in the EEG while the symptom is present and their disappearance as the symptom abates. While this criterion has been fulfilled for certain obtunded states (Goldensohn and Gold, 1960; Rennick et al., 1969) during which the patient may even be irritable, it has not been unequivocally documented in cases of rage attacks.

At this point, we have to address ourselves, however, to a serious limitation of routine electroencephalography, even when the usual activating procedures of hyperventilation, photic stimulation, sleep, and sleep deprivation are used. Pharmacologic activation has been rightfully abandoned for the most part by experts in the profession because of too many false-positive results. We need to remember that our recording electrodes sample mainly the activity of the upper convexity of the cerebral cortex. Mesial surface, orbital frontal, basal temporal, and island of Reil areas as well as the deep structures of the brain are essentially inaccessible to scalp electroencephalography. Attempts are being made to reach the orbital frontal areas through nasopharyngeal electrodes (which tend to be uncomfortable and frequently produce artifact, especially when the patient moves, which is unavoidable during an attack regardless of its nature) and the basal temporal areas through sphenoidal electrodes. Since the latter procedure is an intrusive one, it can be used in only certain specialized centers. The problem is complicated further by the fact that certain pathological electrical events can remain extremely circumscribed, and unless the recording electrode is in the immediate vicinity of the discharging area the pathologic process may remain undetected. For these reasons it is necessary that electrodes are introduced directly into the brain covering those target areas that are involved in the elaboration of behavior, namely, the limbic system, in order to get a clear picture of the function of the structures when the patient is quiet or behaves spontaneously in an agitated manner. Early investigations by Delgado and Hamlin (1956), Sem-Jacobsen et al. (1955), Bickford (1956), and Heath (1962) established quite clearly the complexity of depth electrographic abnormalities, even in the resting state in epileptic and to some extent in psychotic patients. They also showed that specific behavioral responses could be obtained from electrical stimulation of certain deep structures and that epileptic attacks could start in the depth of the brain without being reflected on the surface. In addition, it was demonstrated that the clinical accompaniments could occur prior to the spread of the deep discharges to the scalp EEG. Heath and co-workers demonstrated that when spike wave discharges were limited to the hippocampus and amygdala in an epileptic patient with behavioral disturbances, the patient showed minimal psychotic behavior and when the patient was actively hallucinating, the spike wave discharges became markedly intensified, spreading also to the septal area. The scalp EEG remained normal, however (Heath and Mickle, 1960). It is also important to point out that the patient's behavioral disturbances, consisting of agitation, rage and psychotic thinking, lasted much longer than do most epileptic seizures: hours to days, rather than minutes. Although Mark and Ervin (1970) have also described a seizure discharge in the depths of the brain being associated with rage reaction (patient Julia S.), it resulted from electrical stimulation of the amygdala and it could be argued that it was, therefore, not necessarily representative of the patient's spontaneous episode. One other case of Mark and Ervin, namely, that of the child murderess, must be mentioned because she did not have clinical epilepsy. This was an adolescent girl who twice murdered other children and was intolerant of hearing a baby cry. After depth electrodes had been implanted, a taped recording of a crying baby was played, and " ... a marked behavioral response of discomfort and anxiety ... " as well as anger accompanied by a seizure-like electrical discharge in the depth of the temporal lobe was elicited. Although there was no physical aggression, one must agree that there was a dysphoric response elicited by an essentially normal stimulus in a patient who did not have clinical epilepsy. The only other case of goal directed aggression during depth electrography this reviewer is aware of is a case reported by Saint-Hilaire et al. (1981).

LITERATURE REVIEW OF INDIVIDUAL CASE REPORTS

There are many case reports of violent behavior attributed to seizures (Meyer, 1957; Benay, 1961; Stevenson, 1963; Winfield and Ozturk, 1959; Rabending, 1961). Critical review of documented cases of epilepsy with episodic undesirable behavior reveals either 1) simple confusional states with relatively innocent behavior, 2) confusional states complicated by alcohol ingestion and associated with either relatively innocent or criminal behavior, 3) nonconfusional excessive violence in individuals with chronic anger and excessive irritability, or 4) accidental homicide. Few case reports really qualify as evidence of "ictal violence." Some could be regarded as postictal behavior, but the majority must be viewed as having occurred in the interictal period. While the patients reported in the mentioned references did have epilepsy, there exist several additional reports in which the crime itself is taken as evidence for a seizure disorder (Asuni, 1969; Brewer, 1971).

The confusion that exists in the minds of some "expert" witnesses is probably best documented in the trial transcripts of Robert Torsney and Jack Ruby, who killed President Kennedy's assassin in full view of the nation's TV cameras. Torsney, a police officer, shot at point-blank range and killed a black adolescent who merely inquired if the officer had come from a specified apartment where there had been a civil disturbance. For both Ruby and Torsney, epilepsy was used as a defense in spite of the fact that neither defendant had ever had epileptic seizures, although both had suffered head injuries and had experienced episodic disturbances that could qualify for the "borderland of epilepsy." While Ruby's electroencephalogram, according to the testimony given by Gibbs and members of his school, showed the psychomotor variant type pattern, that of Torsney was according to the trial transcript interpreted as having been normal. Terms like "psychomotor epilepsy," "psychomotor variant epilepsy," "rupture of the ego in a period of episodic dyscontrol," "psychosis associated with epilepsy," "automatism by Penfield (sic)" and others were all used indiscriminately by lawyers and expert witnesses alike in these trials. There are, however, some other interesting parallels in the 2 cases. Both defendants had been brutalized by their alcoholic fathers in childhood, and in both instances the suggestion of epilepsy was initially raised not by a psychiatrist or a neurologist but on the basis of psychological test results. The only psychologic test which directly measures the "paroxysmal drive" was developed by Szondi, but it is not used to any great extent in this country and was not given to these two individuals. The diagnosis was apparently made on the basis of the Rorschach test. According to Delay and Lemperiere (1958), a combination of "organic" and "neurotic" elements in a given protocol raises the question of epilepsy. This view, however, is not shared by psychologists who have extensive experience with epileptic patients and seems to be derived largely from an institutionalized patient population which is not representative of the total spectrum of epilepsy patients. As an aside on the system of criminal justice existing at this time in the United States, it might be mentioned that Ruby was sentenced to life in prison and Torsney was declared not guilty by reason of insanity. The diagnosis of epilepsy was dropped by the defense later during the trial.

NUMERICAL PERSPECTIVE

Having reviewed individual cases, one is struck by the paucity of well-documented goal-directed criminal acts committed by epileptic patients in an ictal or postictal state. It is, therefore, necessary to look at studies that are not anecdotal in nature but statistical. Since the original investigations by Gunn, which are summarized in his book (1977), it is apparent that the prevalence of epileptic patients in prisons is higher than in a general population. Gunn's study initially revealed a rate of 8.8/1000. A more refined technique subsequently revealed a prevalence rate of 7.2/1000, which is still substantially higher than that encountered in the review of general practices in England and Wales by Pond and Bidwell (1960). Novick et al. (1977), studying 1420 prisoners admitted to New York City correctional facilities during a 2 week period in June 1975, found a rate of 3.9% for antiepileptic medications. King and Young (1978), surveying prescription rates for Illinois prison and jail inmates, found a point prevalence of 1.9%. A similar study in North Carolina (Department of Human Resources, 1977) yielded a rate of 1.8%. While these figures are substantially higher than would be expected from the general population, they are potentially misleading because the prison population, especially in the United States, contains a large number of inmates with drug or alcohol problems and some of the seizures may be due to withdrawal states. Another complicating factor is that this group of people as a whole contains an overrepresentation of head injuries and lowered I.Qs which may have resulted from cerebral insults. In addition, the possibility of pseudoseizures also has to be considered. A direct relationship between criminal behavior and epilepsy cannot, therefore, be established on the basis of this type of statistics. The series of studies by Gunn is actually the most exhaustive and, in view of the alleged greater violence that is to be found among patients with temporal lobe seizures, it was revealing to note that not only was there no statistical difference in the degree of violence between epileptic and nonepileptic prisoners but also there was no difference in regard to seizure type within the epilepsy population which was violent. The temporal lobe group had more previous convictions; the "subcortical" group had a larger share of convictions for violence, with the "other focal" seizure group showing a proportionately smaller share. Within the entire English prison system, there were only three individuals who, within 12 hours before or after the offense, had a definite epileptic seizure leading to admission to Broadmore Hospital; two of the three committed their antisocial acts, in all probability, during an altered state of consciousness. One, during an epileptic seizure, struck an elderly male friend with whom he was visiting and who died from the resultant fall. The other developed a seizure after an evening of shooting pigeons; the following morning while still in a confused state, he arose early, took his shotgun and went outside, brandishing the gun in a village street and firing shots occasionally—fortunately no one was hurt.

Korbar and Berkovic (1974), who examined the problem of epilepsy and delinquency in Serbia, found a low socioeconomic stratum as the most significant variable and 83% showed intellectual limitations. Psychomotor epilepsy was present in only 25% and, in all instances, was combined with grand mal seizures. In no case was a crime committed during a seizure, although four delinquent acts were apparently committed during a confusional state. In contrast to Gunn's findings, crimes involving bloodshed occurred in 30% of the average delinquent population but in 46.7% of the epilepsy group. Whether or not this difference is statistically significant could not be ascertained from the data presented and there was no further information as to type of "bloodshed." Ritzel and Ritter (1973) found a conviction rate of 1.5% in epileptic patients attending an outpatient clinic of the university hospital in Goettingen, Germany. Although higher than in the general population, the offenses were exclusively committed by those patients who had concomitant psychiatric disorders. There was no predilection for a given type of offense nor for a specific seizure type. Psychomotor epilepsy was not overrepresented. However, traffic offenses were more serious, with every other one involving bodily injury. Somasundaram (1972) examined 115 criminally mentally ill patients at the government hospital in Madras and found 15 who had epilepsy. All had tonic-clonic seizures. EEGs were obtained in 13 of them: 5 were normal, "centrencephalic" abnormalities occurred in 7, and a temporal focus was noted in 1. A direct relationship between seizures and the criminal acts was not established. Okasha et al. (1975) found 2 epileptic patients among 60 Egyptian murderers; the rest were diagnosed as psychopathic, mentally deficient and schizophrenic, in descending order. Hemmi (1967) conducted a psychiatric study of epileptic patients among habitual offenders in Tokyo Fukue Prison and found 95 cases between 1954 and 1957. He divided the population into a nuclear group (n 20) who had grand mal or petit mal but little or no psychomotor seizures and a peripheral group (n 32) who had grand mal or petit mal and psychomotor seizures and a positive family history of epilepsy. The largest subgroup (n 43) was termed "epileptoid" and had transitory mental symptoms; the patients were otherwise similar to the "peripheral group" but had no personal or family history of grand mal seizures. Violent offenses occurred in 20% of the nuclear group and in 25% of the peripheral group and were "frequent" in the epileptoid group. Alcohol abuse and pathologic drunkenness were among the most frequent precipitants of criminal acts.

Reviewing these aspects of the material, one must conclude that while epileptic patients may intermittently show violent behavior a direct link between a murderous act and an epileptic attack is extremely uncommon, especially if accidental killing is excepted.

VIOLENCE AND AGGRESSION WORKSHOP

The professional advisory board of the Epilepsy Foundation of America has appointed a special committee on epilepsy and violent/aggressive behavior. As part of the effort to generate reliable data, a workshop was held on this topic during March of 1980 in Bethesda, Maryland. Investigators from the United States, Canada, Federal Republic of West Germany and Japan participated. It consisted essentially of viewing 33 videomonitored seizures which were regarded as showing violent behavior. The videotapes that were used resulted from a request by the chairman of the workshop to major epilepsy programs around the world to provide documentation of ictal aggressive behavior. The participants were given a checklist to fill out for each attack as to severity of violent behavior, mood of the individual, type of attack and degree of restraint. The definitions for behavior rating were as follows: 1) Nondirected motor activity—stereotyped nondirected movements such as kicking, flailing, boxing, hitting postures and acts that are not directed to objects or persons in the immediate environment; 2) Violence to property—an act using physical force in a destructive manner toward an inanimate object or an animal; 3) Threatening violence to a person—an act using physical force toward another person and yet not amounting to physical harm. This includes gestures, spitting, shouting; 4) Mild to moderate violence to a person—an act using physical force toward another person without inflicting significant bodily harm; 5) Moderate violence to a person—an act using physical force toward another person and yet not amounting to severe and grievous bodily harm; 6) Severe violence to a person—an act using physical force toward another person, damaging or seriously endangering life or health. The results of the workshop will appear in a separate publication by the members of the committee and, therefore, are not reported in detail here, but this author could not classify even one attack as rating a number 6 on the behavior scale. The maximum consensus rating was a 4 (for only 1 patient) and the total group of collaborators gave mean ratings ranging from 0 to 4, the overall mean rating of the 33 seizures being 1.3. Since the committee will issue its final report later in 1981, further comment is not needed at this time because the facts speak for themselves.

PERSONAL EXPERIENCES

Since its inception in 1959, the neurology program of Lafayette Clinic under the direction of this author has been devoted for the most part to the treatment of epileptic patients. Between 1959 and 1976, 20 beds were available; the unit was enlarged to 42 beds in January 1977. In spite of the fact that the most up-to-date medical, psychiatric and psychologic treatment modalities were available, we saw between 1977 and the summer of 1980, when the program had to be terminated, no less than 4000 seizures per year in our inpatient population. Because Lafayette Clinic was a referral center to which intractable patients from the community and the state mental hospital system were being sent for treatment, this number represented an irreducible minimum with the currently available treatment modalities. Each patient's treatment program was supervised by myself to ensure that optimal care was rendered. The mentioned figure has remained essentially stable over the past 3 years, during which 42 beds were available. It was approximately half of that when the unit consisted of 20 beds. Since complex partial seizures and atonic, tonic, and akinetic seizure types are least responsive to medical treatment, these groups form the largest percentages. Inasmuch as the psychiatric literature continues to point to the dangerous nature of patients with psychomotor epilepsy or, to use the international classification, complex partial seizures, it needs to be stated that, on the average, about one third of the seizures observed on our wards were associated with automatic behavior, either as an ictal or postictal event. Over the mentioned time span of 21 years, we have observed somewhat more than 10,000 epileptic seizures with automatic components. If one uses the definition and adopts the scale as developed for the previously mentioned workshop on aggression and violence as "directed exertion of physical force so as to injure, abuse or destroy," we did not have a single case in our entire material that could be rated as number 6. It must be reemphasized that I was in continuous charge of the program and any serious assault would have had to be brought to my attention. Moderate violence to a person (rating number 5) was seen in less than 10 instances at maximum. Actually, only 3 cases come to mind: 1) An adolescent with a fierce temper suddenly jumped up and hit another patient, who had shown aggravating behavior, over the head with a chair and then calmly sat down again. When asked why he had done it, he replied, "God told me so." 2) An elderly lady, while in a postictal psychotic state, swung her belt at me because she regarded me as the devil. 3) This instance deserves more extensive description because it occurred during an EEG recording and bears considerable resemblance to the patient reviewed by the collaborative study of ictal violence. The incident reports, as filed by the EEG technician and the treating physician, read as follows:

> Patient was received on time for a two o'clock appointment. The patient was friendly and commented on the fact that he had not seen me for quite some time. I asked the patient how he had been doing and he remarked "not too good." He complained of sleeping difficulties and unemployment.

When I asked him about his medication, he replied 'same as always' and when he was asked about how often or how much he took, he was quite vague and finally said "same as before, you know." I proceeded to apply the electrodes. Patient was cooperative throughout and became drowsy as his head bobbed occasionally. When asked if he was tired, he admitted he was.

The EEG was started and proceeded smoothly until shortly after hyperventilation. At this time, the patient opened his eyes, literally jumped out of the chair pulling all the electrodes off, and grabbed the technician by the arm. He kept repeating statements like, "You're coming with me. I'm tired of this. You're under arrest, we're waiting for the big men." He opened the lab door and he and I started down the hall towards the lobby door. I called another technician and she joined us at the door. Patient then pounded on the lobby door and motioned for his mother to join us. When she came, the three of us talked with him, trying to reassure him that he was done and that all we had to do was clean him up. The patient knew his mother and kept insisting that we technicians were going to kill him. We got him back into Room 1210. His mother closed the door and tried talking to him. Patient was extremely agitated and I told the mother to open the door and let him go. The patient then went back into the hallway and yelled "You, come here" and struck the technician. He hit her on the face and her glasses flew off. She slid down the wall and was in a crouched position when he kicked her in the head with his foot.

I don't clearly recall what followed but he turned and clipped my left ear, and grabbed my arm. I went down on the floor, got kicked once in the back and finally someone pulled him away.

(EEG Technician)

The treating physician reported as follows:

This day I had an outpatient appointment with the patient. Patient's mother called me 3 days ago and stated that patient has had a seizure every 20 minutes. That day patient was taken to the Emergency Room at Mt. Clemens Hospital. Patient was released from that hospital. I had a phone call early in the morning of the day of the appointment, and an added EEG appointment was given as well.

In the afternoon I had a phone call from our secretary's office. They mentioned that the patient became violent and they needed my help. I went to the secretary's room and the patient was there. He was surrounded by 3 security guards. I asked one of the guards to bring him to my office. On his way to my office he slid down to the floor and then he said, "I am faking the seizure." Patient was in my office with his mother and for a while patient was quiet. But suddenly patient said to me, "You are the one who wrapped the telephone cord around my neck to kill me." This was calmed down by mother. I let him and the mother wait in my office. I went to the EEG room to look at the EEG. There I was told our EEG technicians were beaten by him. At this point I decided he should be staying in the hospital.

Diagnosis at that time was postictal psychosis or patient took some hard medicine like hallucinogen.

Later I talked with the physician who examined the EEG technicians. He stated he did not find anything wrong with either of them.

Incident was discussed in conference the next morning.

(Physician's signature)

The important aspects are: 1) the attack came on after hyperventilation. In contrast to absence seizures which are precipitated during hyperventilation, our experience has shown that complex partial seizures frequently follow hyperventilation by an interval of 1–2 minutes. 2) The patient did not have any of the classical aspects of a complex partial seizure. There was no chewing, smacking, swallowing, tonic extension of one or both upper extremities, picking or fussing behavior. 3) He remained in contact with his environment, recognized his mother, but mistook the EEG personnel and the physician for personal enemies. 4) Verbalizations were intact and purposeful, considering his psychotic ideation at the time. 5) The attack was unprovoked and self-limited. 6) Although the patient later on stated to the physician that he was "faking a seizure," the attack on the technicians was real and, in my personal opinion, involuntary. 7) Although the EEG record had normalized immediately prior to the incident, it does seem likely that he had indeed an ictal event limited to deep temporal lobe structures on the right side, thus permitting speech, as in cases C.S. and F.F. of Saint-Hilaire and patient H.G. of Heath. Since only scalp electroencephalography was available, this conclusion must remain a reasonable assumption rather than a proven fact.

Apart from these incidents, we did have episodes where patients who had intermittently harmless complex partial seizures ripped up furniture on other occasions; in our best judgment these attacks were not epileptic in nature in spite of having occurred in epileptic patients because the individuals remained in contact with the environment, vented their anger in this fashion and responded to a behavior modification program.

Mark and Ervin (1970) as well as Monroe (1970) have rightfully attacked the unfortunate "either-or" philosophy that dominates thought patterns even of professionals in this country. Briefly stated, if someone has epilepsy, or even only an abnormal electroencephalogram, then all of his abnormal activities may be glibly attributed to epilepsy. If someone has a normal EEG and normal neurological examination and has a mother-in-law whom he hates but cannot get rid of, the resulting depression is considered to be "psychogenic." The prospects that the first individual may fake seizures to get attention or even to hide a criminal act (see Smerdyakov in Dostoveski's *Brothers Karamazov*) or that the second may have a temporal tumor that is too small to appear on a CT scan may be overlooked if a patient's condition is bound to exclusively psychiatric or neurologic interpretations. This fallacy, which has set the field of neuropsychiatry back for decades, must be exposed and abandoned if we really want to understand our patients and to provide appropriate help. The coexistence of epilepsy and psychogenic attacks is not at all rare and occurs in at least one quarter of our admittedly more severely ill epileptic population.

Case Report

The following case report will show the interactions between epileptic, social and psychogenic mechanisms. It also points out that the entire life history of a patient has to be taken into account in order to place a patient's behavior at a given moment into proper perspective.

JRB was first referred for diagnostic purposes to the Epilepsy Center of Michigan in June 1964 by the consulting psychiatrist for the school district the patient was living in. The patient was a 6½-year-old boy who had suffered a nocturnal grand mal seizure at the age of 10½ months. He was taken to a local hospital but it took 2–3 hours before the attack was brought under control. No medications were prescribed and a similar attack occurred during the following week. The seizures were not precipitated by fever or other accompanying illness. Following these major seizures the patient developed minor attacks, consisting of coming to his mother and complaining of stomach difficulties. His lips were pursed tightly and appeared somewhat cyanotic; occasionally there was slurring of speech. At times the patient collapsed to the ground with these episodes. They occurred 3 to 4 times a week but the history noted only one further tonic-clonic seizure, at age 5½ years.

Shortly after the onset of the patient's seizure disorder, he was started on Atarax because of hyperkinetic behavior. Only after the third major seizure was Atarax discontinued and replaced by phenytoin. The mother felt that while the boy was on Atarax, he was much calmer and she did not understand why he was taken off that drug. However, phenytoin did lead to improvement of the minor attacks. His main problem and the reason for referral to the Center was "intolerable behavior in the kindergarten class." He was hyperactive, could not get along with other children, was aggressive, had no sense of danger, could not be contained in quiet activities, even like watching T.V. for any length of time. A pertinent excerpt from the kindergarten teacher, states as follows: "...did much hitting with hands or toys, kicking, pushing and seizing of toys, was restless, paid little attention to the teacher, talking constantly, did not attempt to do the work and was destructive of materials and toys, tearing and/or breaking them. He also threw toys and articles of clothing into the toilet, masturbated frequently, and was involved in running feuds with other children who called him crazy. In the visiting teacher room he was not hostile but moved restlessly about, looked at and touched everything, asked many questions, smiled constantly, was very eager to come and reluctant to go. Insisted he was supposed to stay. He played simple games. The family dolls fought and the parents had intercourse. His speech was free. One day he stumbled over a chair, said 'you dirty son of a bitch' and gave it a kick. He used four-letter words in the course of a conversation without indicating he felt they were bad." Past medical history of the child was otherwise negative.

Family History: One maternal uncle and aunt stillborn; father had small seizures similar to patient's between the ages of 3 and 7.

Social History: The father, an unskilled worker, suffered from severe chronic alcohol abuse and the family was in serious financial difficulties. The mother had recently taken a job to help pay off some of the debts incurred on account of the father's behavior. The mother appeared to be reliable but was quite defensive about the patient. She admitted to being overprotective but minimized the patient's behavioral difficulties, felt that his rejection by others was unjustifiable. She had been told about her overprotectiveness and that the patient had improved even in the short time when she was away from home working. Although she professed to be anxious to know what she was doing wrong, she found it hard to accept that her feelings toward the patient may have been detrimental. The clinical neurological examination was negative. So were the routine laboratory tests and the electroencephalogram. On psychiatric evaluation, the patient was noted to be well developed and well nourished but dressed rather carelessly in inexpensive soiled clothing. The shirt, mostly unbuttoned, was hanging out of his pants, hair was unkempt, fingernails were dirty. When the psychiatrist called him into the interviewing room, the patient was piling up checkers in a long train and although he heard the call he did not come until he finished what he was doing and said under his breath, "I am going to finish this first." He seemed alert but spoke quite rapidly and at times it was difficult to understand him. Intellectual limitations were obvious. He was unable to print his name and could not understand why his printing was wrong even after the correct way had been shown to him. When asked what the father did, expecting an answer as to occupation, the boy replied that his father whipped him and the other children were always telling on him. Although he was able to remain in the chair during the interview, he was restless, fidgety, sometimes talking in a very loud and at other times in a very soft voice and there was a tendency to perseverate. On psychological testing, the same type of behavior was observed. He frequently used the word "shit" without being disturbed by it. On formal testing, he achieved a Stanford-Binet I.Q. of 77. In addition, it was felt that he had serious brain dysfunction, more marked on the left. The psychiatrist and psychologist agreed that the patient was not amenable to psychother-apy and that he should be placed on medication, either amphetamines or tranquilizers. In addition, he should receive education in a special classroom. The parents were advised to seek help at the local family service society.

In April 1970, at age 12, he was seen by myself. There had been no change since the age of 6. He still had stomachaches, and he also complained of headaches and got excited very easily. The headaches were located on the right side in the parietal area; it felt like the head was being squeezed together. They occurred twice a day and lasted 1 or 2 minutes. There had not been any further generalized seizures. Neurological examination was essentially negative but a questionable Babinski sign was noted on the left and could have been a withdrawal response. There was some difficulty hopping on the left leg and clumsiness on rapid alternate motions, more on the left than on the right. The EEG was again negative. The behavior had continued to be unacceptable. He was very disruptive but punishment was totally ineffective. He acted impulsively, argued, fought, felt that he was picked on by everybody else and was not loved, had threatened to run away from home and to kill himself, but had never harmed anybody. Again medical management was advised but so were firm controls, and it was also suggested that the parents must reach an agreement in the handling of the patient. I saw him again in 1971. My note at that time states: "There has been no improvement in the patient's behavior, on the contrary it might even be somewhat worse." There was constant arguing and bickering between the patient and his mother in the office. The boy used all sorts of attention-getting devices and was openly angry, but in a joking manner, and he seemed to derive considerable satisfaction from displaying his anger. He continued to complain of stomachaches but was quite vague in this complaint. He stated that it lasted 3 minutes and it comes twice a day, especially when he goes to sleep. The school had excluded him from next year's program. Attempts were made to get him into a particular special program beyond the special education class he had been in, but it was doubtful that he would be able to be placed. He had an extremely violent temper, had broken his hand on two occasions striking objects as a result of his temper. In view of the severity of the problem I suggested that he be admitted to Lafayette Clinic for evaluation and treatment. At that time his electroencephalogram was no longer negative but showed a sharp wave focus in the left temporal area. During his hospitalization, from 8/16/71 to 9/20/71, he was initially quite uncooperative, tested limits continuously but improved when rules were enforced. No seizures were observed. There were no headaches and no stomachaches. He was discharged on phenytoin, 300 mg, carbamazepine, 800 mg, thioridazine, 150 mg, but had to be readmitted on 2/27/73 to 5/7/73 because of poor seizure control and unacceptable behavior. In the hospital he was again seizure free but argumentative with peers. He started physical fights. Strict enforcement of limits led to improvement. The EEG showed again left temporal sharp discharge and some generalized disorganization. He was discharged on phenytoin, 500 mg, carbamazepine, 800 mg, and phenobarbital, 90 mg.

On May 18, 1977 he was readmitted after he had been discharged from Pontiac State Hospital 2 weeks earlier. He had been hospitalized there off and on for the past 2½ years because of unacceptable behavior, temper tantrums, and having gotten into fights. At Pontiac State Hospital he had knocked another patient's teeth out, shown poor judgment, had gone out in the snow barefoot. The parents had to watch him constantly; they never knew what he would do next. Seizures were now mostly of the psychomotor variety. He would talk irrelevantly, produce high-pitched sounds, and pick at objects and walls. They lasted for 10 to 15 minutes and then he was all right. Episodes recurred several times a week. EEG showed a bitemporal sharp wave focus, maximal on the left. During hospitalization, haloperidol and chlorpromazine were tried in addition to anticonvulsants but were found ineffective in controlling his behavior. The neurologic examination was negative. He ran away twice. During the second time he hitchhiked to Cincinnati and was therefore discharged from the hospital. A CT scan had been performed and had shown some abnormality involving the right frontal area. This could not be followed up because of the patient's having left the center.

In September 1979 he was seen again by myself at the Epilepsy Center, where he was brought because of an increased number of "seizures" during which he became physically violent and aggressive. He picked up objects and threw them around. The attacks occurred several times a day. At night they were preceded by a scream. The patient might fall out of bed and subsequently enter into automatic activities during which he tended to destroy furniture. In the daytime he had a 10 to 5 second warning of stomachache and subsequently engaged in these activities. For instance, the day I saw him he had ripped out the rearview mirror of the car while the mother was driving him to the Center. He had also grabbed the steering wheel. The attacks occurred several times a day as was well as during the night. An attack was observed in the EEG laboratory and the following is a description by the technologist: "The patient was drowsy and sitting in reclined chair with eyes closed. He cried out, sat up, then cried out again, and bounced up from the chair. He grabbed the strobe lamp (mounted on stand), began to swing it and drag it towards the door. Technician held door shut from the outside while patient held lamp in one hand and pulled on door with other. He managed to force his way through the door dragging the strobe, but technician closed door catching the base of the strobe stand between the door and frame. Patient crouched in doorway looking at technician and trying to pull the lamp through and/or push the door open. With the arrival of a second employee, who held onto the strobe lamp (patient still pulling on it), the technician stepped over patient to check the EEG and then in a stern voice asked the patient if he was "finished." Patient said "Uh huh," nodded his head, let go of the strobe stand and stood upright. He wiped his hands on his pants, straightened his hair and, on command, walked back into the EEG lab. Patient stated he felt that he had lost some money in the chair, checked his pockets and then repeated the comment (speech pattern at this point was not smooth). Patient was cooperative, got back into chair, electrodes were reapplied and he fell asleep shortly thereafter. Estimated duration of entire event was 6 minutes. Actual 'seizure' lasted from 2 to 2½ minutes. The EEG did not show seizure discharges during this episode.

The patient at that time was on 500 mg of Dilantin but had a level of only 9.7 μg/ml. Although I felt that the patient was going to produce a profound behavioral disturbance on the ward at the Lafayette Clinic, I had no choice but to readmit him to the Clinic because he would not be treatable on an outpatient basis. I added in my note that he is likely to be untreatable even at Lafayette Clinic, but we can evaluate whether or not he might be eligible for a surgical procedure. At that time I did not have the Lafayette Clinic record available showing the previously abnormal CT scan. I also felt that it was likely that not all of the patient's attacks were indeed epileptic in nature, although the majority seemed to be. He was then admitted to the Clinic where he stayed for 4 weeks. During his hospitalization we immediately imposed firm limits and no major incident occurred. His behavior on the ward was unremarkable except for one occasion when he grabbed a female patient, but this was not seizure related. There were no clinical seizures during hospitalizaton.

Over the years the patient had several psychological evaluations at Lafayette Clinic. The I.Q. was in the borderline range and most of the time he had a significantly higher Performance than Verbal I.Q., indicating left hemisphere dysfunction. Even at the time of his last admission, he was unable to read. In 1974 a significant drop in Performance I.Q. was seen and was regarded as evidence of deterioration, but by 1977 the Performance I.Q. had again risen thus suggesting that the deficit was of a chronic and static nature. Projective tests had always shown severe personality disruption and only the result of the last evaluation in 1979 will be reported here in some detail. "The patient shows inadequate reality testing and poor ego control. His thinking frequently is quite arbitrary as he responds to his internal preoccupations and distorts the reality around him. His thoughts are drained of energy, lifeless and morbid in content. There are paranoid features to his thinking. He sees his environment as threatening and dangerous. He completely denies any feeling of anger or hostility, yet is preoccupied with the unprovoked 'hateful' behavior of others toward him. He feels wronged, mistreated, yet overprotests that he is full of 'love.' He must guard himself from others by constant vigilance and wary watching. Emotionally he is flat and anhedonic, covering this over with a very shallow veneer of affability and good humor. There was also evidence for a morbid sexual confusion, a primitive uncertainty about how men and women differ sexually. He also seems to be guarded and uncomfortable around men, feeling threatened, projecting homosexual concerns onto them and needing to defend himself against possible sexual assault. He is highly ambivalent toward women, attracted yet repelled, fearful, angry and disdainful all at once. Some bizarre or morbid sexual acts, possibly involving violence, seem in character with the pathology seen in this patient. Despite the presence of an underlying thought disorder, the patient is at this time in marginal contact with reality and not clearly psychotic. The patient would be employable except for long-standing psychiatric problems and the presence

                                        205

of seizures. Prognosis for treatment by psychotherapy is extremely poor due to patient's lack of insight.

The patient had no seizures or other episodic behavior on the ward. The EEG showed again a left temporal sharp wave focus and a repeat CT scan showed a calcified lesion in the *right* basofrontal temporal area. A low-grade astrocytoma was suspected and surgical exploration recommended. The patient was therefore transferred to Harper-Grace Hospital where a resection of the right anterior temporal lobe was carried out. The histologic examination of the operative specimen showed a vascular malformation of arteriovenous type with degenerative changes and secondary astrocytosis of the brain. On the first postoperative day, I received a call from the Intensive Care Unit at Harper-Grace Hospital and a report that the patient had attempted to choke a nurse. On investigation of the incident it became apparent that the patient was in a confusional state, had had an abortive seizure during which both arms were extended upward and when the nurse leaned over the bed, he clutched her neck tightly, his grip could be loosened by others. The patient was given phenytoin and haloperidol and lapsed into sleep. He had no memory of the event the following day. When seen on that day he was pleasant, claimed that he is a good person who followed the Lord Jesus, and would never harm anybody. He was not psychotic or confused and behaved appropriately consistent with circumstances of an ICU. It was explained to the nursing staff that they must be extremely firm with this patient, not allow the slightest deviation from hospital rules and not show fear but confront him strictly with authority. This regimen was successful and on request of the parents, who did not want to take him home directly after his surgical wound had healed, it was agreed that he could convalesce for an additional 2 or 3 weeks at Lafayette Clinic. While there, with firm limits, again there were neither seizures nor behavioral outbursts. It was our feeling, supported by psychological testing, that the patient was now even more surly, argumentative, impulsive, and showed very poor judgment. Previously he had had, to some degree, a sense of humor which made him, in spite of his problems, likeable to the extent that he had been elected ward president during his preoperative state; he now annoyed the other patients, who did not want to have any dealings with him. Although we felt that this patient was now potentially even more dangerous than he was preoperatively because of total lack of insight, he was not committable under current laws because he had not inflicted grievous bodily harm either to himself or to anyone else. Since he could not be kept at the Clinic for an unlimited period of time, he had to be returned to his reluctant parents.

In conclusion, this case presents the failure of our society to deal with a mixed social, neurologic and psychiatric problem occurring in the same individual. It can be argued that if the 6-year-old had not been brutalized by his father and overindulged by his mother, he might have grown into an individual with dull-normal intelligence who would have performed simple manual labor although he might have had occasional minor seizures. These would have, however, readily responded to anticonvulsant medications as his repeated hospitalizations proved. Had the parents imposed the limits that were set in the hospital, there would likewise not have been major behavioral problems. Although the patient's primary pathology was left-sided (initial EEG focus on the left, low verbal I.Q. and complete dyslexia), he had independent, possibly neoplastic disease on the right which required surgical exploration. Whatever positive features the right anterior temporal lobe contributed to the patient's personality were compromised by surgery and he was left with his original pathology compounded by an even greater lack of judgment. We are now confronted with an individual who may well commit a serious act of violence resulting in either a prison sentence or, as our psychologist suggested, the patient may irritate others sufficiently to become the victim of a barroom brawl with potentially serious injury or even fatal outcome for the patient. Since our society demands a victim before correctional steps can be taken, the physician has to stand by and let fate take over. Assuming that a criminal act will be committed, which might have happened had the patient been alone with the nurse, he probably would under those circumstances have been adjudged as not guilty by reason of insanity and sent to a state mental institution. It is also likely he would be free again under our current system within a matter of a few months or a few years maximally, because he functions well in a controlled environment. The United States has at this time neither programs nor plans for such that would allow the humane removal of individuals from society who cannot function by themselves and will never be able to do so.

NEUROPHYSIOLOGIC THEORY AND SUGGESTIONS FOR FUTURE RESEARCH

It appears clear that there exist a group of people liable to criminal behavior, but who are not readily found among the common EEG or neurological classifications. The opinion expressed by Lorimer (1977) in a roundtable discussion on violent behavior and the electroencephalogram is probably correct: " . . . there exists in some people who commit acts of violence a medical condition of malfunction of the brain—particularly the limbic systems—that is as much a medical disease as is diabetes." The symptoms of this "disease" were described as follows: headaches, spells usually not typically epileptic in nature and personality change. The underlying etiology must remain speculative at this time and, as in the Ruby and Torsney transcripts, probably consists of a mixture of organic and psychosocial factors. Nevertheless, it may be useful to delineate the difference between "epileptic" and "epileptoid" within a theoretical neurophysiologic framework. Epilepsy, according to the currently accepted definition which goes back to Hughlings Jackson, is "a sudden excessive discharge of gray matter." To this should be added, as this author has pointed out previously (1972), the qualifying statement: " . . . which spreads to other parts of the CNS and usually the musculature." Not only the site of origin of the discharge but also the speed of spread determines whether a grand mal seizure will be regarded clinically as of focal or nonfocal onset. If spread occurs within a matter of several seconds, the attack will be regarded as having a focal origin; if spread occurs within a few milliseconds, the seizure will be regarded as nonfocal or, in the international terminology, primary generalized. It can now be hypothesized that, while speed of spread which depends on the interplay of excitatory and inhibitory forces within the brain determines focal versus nonfocal, extent of spread and duration of discharge determine whether an attack is regarded as epileptic or "epileptoid" or whatever name, like "masked epilepsy," "epileptic equivalent," or "episodic dyscontrol," one may want to choose. It is readily conceivable that there may be certain patients whose neurotransmitter system is so composed that both an excess of excitation and inhibition exist at given times, producing thereby the clinical picture of a person who experiences that something is going wrong but who has such a high threshold for spread of abnormal excitation that a clinically recognizable epileptic seizure will not result. The commonly quoted statement that anybody can have an epileptic seizure given sufficient amounts of electricity to his brain, thereby suggesting "you too can have epilepsy and it is nothing to be ashamed of," is only partially valid. Every psychiatrist who has given electroconvulsive treatments knows that great differences in threshold exist and while insulin shock treatment was still being given, it was also clear that although some individuals convulsed, others did not.

I was especially impressed by 1 patient who had committed a seemingly motiveless murder by shooting in systematic fashion his wife and children, but before shooting himself he called the police. He claimed amnesia for the act and the crime was apparently motiveless. I saw this man in Jackson prison in 1956 and since in the 1950s justified medical research could still proceed without legal complications, we obtained first a routine electroencephalogram which was negative. I subsequently tried to induce an attack by means of pentylenetetrazol because the patient had complained of having suffered from previous blackouts, without, however, ever having harmed anyone. I was at that time engaged in trying to establish the usefulness of the method for diagnostic purposes in the practice of psychiatry and had had considerable experience with the drug. To my surprise, even after 2000 mg of pentylene-tetrazol—a dose I had never given before and I have not given since—the subject had neither electroencephalographic seizure discharges nor a clinical attack. He did become extremely uncomfortable but remained cooperative. Whether his extremely high threshold had any bearing on his criminal act remains, of course, unanswerable. This man had a great deal of remorse over his crime, which he himself could not understand, and he subsequently committed suicide in jail. It is readily conceivable that such people have episodic electroencephalographic alterations in the depth of the brain which remain very localized, do not reach motor centers and by being partial rather than diffuse can last minutes to hours rather than seconds or minutes, as is the case with the usual epileptic seizures. The use of antiepileptic drugs for sudden inexplicable attacks of violence is controversial. Although some authors, especially Monroe (1970), who share these ideas feel that anticonvulsant medication can be helpful in these cases, my own experience does not tend to bear this out. We simply have too many clearly epileptic patients who are on anticonvulsants, like JRB, and who also have profound dysphoric components to their illness with subsequent intermittent undesirable behavior. If the assumption of *limited spread* of ictal discharge underlying these behaviors is correct, one could even expect a negative result on theoretical grounds, because most current anticonvulsant medications limit spread rather than abolishing a focal irritative process. This might also account for the observation that some epileptic patients do become behaviorally worse on anticonvulsant medications and improve when seizures recur as a result of medication reduction. On the other hand, there are many reports of undesirable episodic nonepileptic behavior in epileptic individuals improving after temporal lobectomy. As Gibbs and Gibbs (1963) have pointed out, the area of "epileptoid" behavior is indeed a morass, but I am personally convinced that it will, in all probability, not be solved by surface electroencephalography. In the present state of technology, only depth electrography is capable of giving reasonable answers, although in the future, positron scanners and nuclear magnetic resonators might become useful noninvasive techniques for the study of these phenomena. While such studies, and others dealing with hormonal environments, are not yet feasible, greater attention should be given to the role of alcohol in precipitating some "motiveless" violent crimes. The pathophysiology of "pathological intoxication" is far from clear but clinical experience shows that some patients who have suffered a moderate degree of brain damage become intolerant to small doses of alcohol, sometimes with catastrophic consequences which not often are clearly related to epileptic mechanisms.

THE MEDICOLEGAL DILEMMA AND RECOMMENDATIONS FOR "EXPERT WITNESS" TESTIMONY

The changes in social climate during the 1970s have made justified medical research with patients who have committed serious antisocial acts, for all practical purposes, impossible. A Detroit court—as a result of this author's attempt to bring some scientific light into the existing confusion—ruled that prisoners or inmates of state institutions cannot under any circumstances give voluntary informed consent to medical research into the causes of their behavior, especially if the research involves depth electrography. The reason given was that it violates the patient's rights under the 1st Amendment to the Constitution of the United States which protects "the generation and free flow of ideas from unwarranted interference with one's mental processes." The human rights of prisoners to have the causes of their behavior explored and, if possible, remedied are, therefore, being denied in the name of protecting their human rights to the integrity of their thinking—regardless of how aberrant and destructive to the person himself his thinking may be and regardless of the patient's desire to have these investigations performed. Much has been written about the "Detroit Psychosurgery Trial," but the medical facts surrounding the patient were not admitted in evidence at the court hearing so as not to jeopardize the patient's adjustment in society. They have never been published and cannot safely be published even now without the risk of further litigation. This is the case in spite of the fact that if this material were to be made public it would shed a considerably different light on the situation than was presented in the judge's opinion. As a result, conscientious scientists are simply staying away from patients of this type and the legal profession has succeeded in stopping constructive research in this area for the time being.

Given our current state of ignorance on the biological aspects of criminal behavior and given the fact that significant inroads will not be made in this country in the foreseeable future, what services can and should the expert witness render when epilepsy is used as a defense strategy? The physician is faced with a dual responsibility under these circumstances, namely, 1) to the defendant and 2) to all other epileptic patients who are law-abiding citizens. It is ill-advised to make an epilepsy defense on tenuous grounds because epileptic patients still have a considerable stigma to bear and they simply do not need this type of unwarranted publicity. In order to avoid the spectacle of competing mutually contradictory expert witnesses in litigation in which the diagnosis of epilepsy is raised, a nationally known and respected epileptologist (possibly recommended through the American Epilepsy Society) should be asked to give testimony as a friend of the court rather than for the defense or prosecution. This expert witness would then establish, on the basis of his interview with the patient and, where applicable, members of the family and other witnesses: 1) whether or not the patient has ever suffered from any of the recognized forms of epilepsy; 2) if a seizure disorder has been present, whether it is currently active or has been in remission for several years; 3) whether the type of seizure the patient habitually has is of a nature that could conceivably lead to a criminal act; 4) whether the criminal act was related in time—either preceding or following—to one of the patient's typical seizures, and 5) whether the patient was obtunded preceding or during the event. In order to hold the patient innocent on account of epilepsy, all of these criteria and not just one would have to be met. It is inadmissible to use the crime itself as evidence for epilepsy, regardless of how bizarre the circumstances. If these five criteria cannot be met, but the EEG is abnormal and/or the patient had shown "epileptoid" traits, the expert witness would simply have to admit that we are at the limits of current medical knowledge and research is required to establish the potential biological factors underlying this condition.

In order to avoid the problem of having to choose between state mental hospitals (which have no cures for most patients) and prisons (which are likewise unproductive), special facilities may have to be created for these unfortunate individuals where they can spend their lives in a human and productive environment but with the imposition of behavioral limits. This would remove them from the pressures and temptations of living in a competitive society which, by nature of their physiology and upbringing, they are unable to tolerate. I realize that this sounds utopian and regressive, going contrary to the current vogue of integrating everyone into society in the name of community psychiatry, but, just as we have to isolate patients with typhoid fever to prevent the spread of infection, we need to take appropriate measures to protect potential victims from acts for which the assailant may actually not carry full responsibility.

References

Asuni, T. Homicide in Western Nigeria. *Br. J. Psychiatry* 115:1105–1113, 1969.

Benay, R.S. Criminal genesis and the degree of responsibility in epilepsies. *Am. J. Psychiatry* 117:873–876, 1961.

Bickford, R.G. The application of depth electrography in some varieties of epilepsy. *EEG Clin. Neurophysiol.* 8:526–527, 1956.

Brewer, C. Homicide during a psychomotor seizure. *Med. J. Aust.* 1:857–859, 1971.

Delay, P., and Lemperiere, P. *The Rorschach and the Epileptic Personality.* Logo Press, New York, 1958.

Delgado, J.M.R., and Hamlin, H. Surface and depth electrography of the frontal lobes in conscious patients. *EEG Clin. Neurophysiol 8:*371–384, 1956.

Epilepsy in North Carolina: Resources and Recommendations. Raleigh, NC, Chronic Disease Branch, Department of Human Resources, August 1977.

Gibbs, F., and Gibbs, E. *Atlas of Electroencephalography, Vol. 2, Epilepsy.* Addison/Wesley Press, Inc., Cambridge, MA, 1952.

Gibbs, F., and Gibbs, E. Borderland of epilepsy. *J. Neuropsychiatr. 4:*287–295, 1963.

Gibbs, F., and Gibbs, E. Fourteen and six per second positive spikes. *EEG Clin. Neurophysiol. 15:*553–558, 1963.

Goldensohn, E., and Gold, A. Prolonged behavioral disturbances as ictal phenomena. *Neurology 10:*1–9, 1960.

Gunn, J. *Epileptics in Prison.* Academic Press, New York, 1977.

Heath, R.G. Common characteristics of epilepsy and schizophrenia: Clinical observation and depth electrode studies. *Am. J. Psychiatry 118:*1013–1026, 1962.

Heath, R.G., and Mickle, W.A. Evaluation of 7 years' experience in human patients. In *Electrical Studies on Unanesthetized Brain,* edited by Ramey, E.R., and O'Doherty, D.S. Hoeber Publishers, New York, 1960.

Hemmi, T. A psychiatric study on epileptics among habitual offenders. *Osaka Ika Daigaku, Bull. Suppl. 12:*379–384, 1967.

Hill, D., and Watterson, D. Electro-encephalographic studies of psychopathic personalities. *J. Neurol. Psychiatry 5:*47–65, 1942.

Hughes, J., Schlagenhauff, R., and Magoss, M. Electro-clinical correlations in the six per second spike and wave complex. *EEG Clin. Neurophysiol. 18:*71–77, 1965.

Jackson, J.H. On temporary mental disorders after epileptic paroxysms. In *Selected Writings of John Hughlings Jackson. vol. I, On Epilepsy and Epileptiform Convulsions,* edited by Taylor, J. Staples Press, London, 1958.

King, L.N., and Young, Q.D. Increased prevalence of seizure disorders among prisoners. *J.A.M.A. 239:*2674–2675, 1978.

Korbar, K., and Berkovic, K. Epilepsy and delinquency. *Neuropshijatirja 22:*61–75, 1974.

Lombroso-Ferrero, G. *Criminal Man According to the Classification of Cesare Lombroso.* Publication No. 134: Patterson Smith Reprint Series in Criminology, Law Enforcement, and Social Problems. Patterson Smith, Montclair, NJ, 1972.

Lorimer, F.M. (Panel Member). American Medical Electroencephalographic Association. Roundtable Discussion: Violent Behavior and the Electroencephalogram. New Orleans, LA, May 1972. *Clin. EEG 3:*180–214, 1972.

Mark, V.H., and Ervin, F.R. *Violence and the Brain.* Harper & Row, New York, 1970.

Maudsley, H. *Responsibility in Mental Disease.* New York, 1874.

Meyer, J.E. Zur Forensischen Bedeutung der Temporallappen-Epilepsie. *Dtsch. Z. Ges. Gerichtl. Med. 46:*212–225, 1957.

Monroe, R. *Episodic Behavioral Disorders.* Harvard University Press, Cambridge, MA, 1970.

Nassi, A.J., and Abramowitz, S.I. From phrenology to psychosurgery and back again: Biological studies of criminality. *Am. J. Orthopsychiatry 46:*591–607, 1976.

Novick, L. F., Penna, R.D., Schwartz, M.S., et al. Health status of the New York City prison population. *Med. Care 15:*205–216, 1977.

Okasha, A., Sadek, A., and Moneim, S.A. Psychosocial and electroencephalographic studies of Egyptian murderers. *Br. J. Psychiatry 126:*34–40, 1975.

Pond, D.A., and Bidwell, B.H. A survey of epilepsy in fourteen general practices: II. Social and psychological aspects. *Epilepsia 1:*285–299, 1960.

Rabending, G. Zur forensischen Psychiatrie der Psychomotorischen Epilepsie. *Psychiatr. Neurol. Med. Psychol. 13:*17–23, 1961.

Rennick, P.M., Perez-Borja, C., and Rodin, E.A. Transient mental deficits associated with recurrent prolonged epileptic clouded state. *Epilepsia 10:*397–405, 1969.

Riley, T.L., and Niedermeyer, E. Rage attacks and episodic violent behavior: Electroencephalographic findings and general considerations. *Clin. EEG 9:*131–138, 1978.

Ritzel, G., and Ritter, G. Neue Ergebnisse zur Kriminalitat von Epileptikern. *Beitr. Gerichtl. Med.* 31:79–86, 1973.

Rodin, E.A. Medical and social prognosis in epilepsy. *Epilepsia* 13:121–131, 1972.

Saint-Hilaire, J.M., Gilbert, M., Bouvier, G., et al. Epilepsy and aggression. In *Epilepsy Updated: Its Causes and Treatment.* Symposia Specialists, Inc., Miami, in press.

Schwade, E.D., and Geiger, S.G. Matricide with electroencephalographic evidence of thalamic or hypothalamic disorder. *Dis. Nerv. Syst.* 14:18–20, 1953.

Sem-Jacobsen, C.W., Petersen, M., Lazarte, J., et al. Electroencephalographic rhythms from the depths of the frontal lobe in 60 psychotic patients. *EEG Clin. Neurophysiol. 7:* 193–210, 1955.

Silverman, D. Clinical and electroencephalographic studies on criminal psychopaths. *Arch. Neurol. Psychiatry* 50:18–33, 1943.

Somasundaram, O. Crimes of persons with epilepsy. *Indian J. Psychiat.* 14:423–435, 1972.

Stafford-Clark, D., and Taylor, F.H. Clinical and electro-encephalographic studies of prisoners charged with murder. *Neurosurg. Psychiatry* 12:325–330, 1949.

Stevenson, H.G. Psychomotor epilepsy associated with criminal behavior. *Med. J. Aust.* 50:784–785, 1963.

Tempkin, O. *The Falling Sickness.* Johns Hopkins Press, Baltimore, 1971.

Tippett, D.L., and Pine, I. Denial mechanisms in masked epilepsy. *Psychosom. Med. 19:* 326–331, 1957.

Turner, W.A. *Epilepsy: A Study of the Idiopathic Disease.* Raven Press, New York, 1973.

Walker, A.E. Murder or epilepsy? *J. Nerv. Ment. Dis.* 133:430–437, 1961.

Winfield, D.L., and Ozturk, O. Electroencephalographic findings in matricide. *Dis. Nerv. Syst.* 20:176–178, 1959.

 # Legal Aspects of Pseudoseizures

THOMAS G. GUTHEIL, M.D.
MARK J. MILLS, J.D., M.D.

> The physician will leave it to the jurist to construct a responsibility that is artificially limited to the metapsychological ego. It is notorious that the greatest difficulties are encountered by attempts to derive from such a construction any practical consequences not in contradiction to human feelings (Freud, 1925).

Psychiatrist and jurist have struggled with each other's constructions in many areas beside the one with which Freud was concerned, the question of responsibility for "immoral" dream content. The complexities of the ambiguous term "responsibility" in this context are reviewed by Moore (1979) in his detailed discussion of responsibility for actions motivated by unconscious determinants. Nonepileptic seizures pose a similar perplexity for clinicolegal understanding. This chapter will examine some of those perplexities and offer the clinician some approaches to the legal issues involved in treating patients with those disorders.

HISTORICAL PERSPECTIVE

Nearly a century ago, the student wishing to learn about hysterical seizures would have gravitated naturally to Charcot at the Salpêtrière. Yet without the student's knowledge (or, for that matter, without Charcot's knowledge) the authenticity of the data he/she would study lay under a cloud of doubt.

The phenomena in question were described by Charcot in this manner:

> The patient loses consciousness and the *paroxysm* proper begins...the patient executes certain epileptiform convulsive movements ... great gesticulations of salutation which are of extreme violence, interrupted from

> time to time by an arching of the body which is absolutely characteristic ... the patient utters wild cries ... the delirium and hallucinations still continue for some time ... the attack is over, although it is generally sure to be repeated a few minutes later ... never during the course of these crises has he bitten his tongue or wet his bed (Charcot, 1888).

The observational skills of this great clinician, no matter how confident of validity (note the remark, "absolutely characteristic"), soon fell under the shadow of skepticism. Havens (1973) notes:

> The young hysterics, living in the Salpêtrière, held the epileptics when they fell and nursed them during their post-seizure confusion.... "In 1899, about six years after Charcot's death," wrote one of his successors, "I saw as a young intern the old patients of Charcot who were still hospitalized. Many of the women, who were excellent comediennes, when they were offered a slight pecuniary remuneration, imitated perfectly the major hysteric crises of former times." ... Janet was to argue that suggestibility was a more reliable sign of hysteria than anesthesia or attacks and that this very suggestibility allowed the patients to be molded to the clinic's expectations.

Thus, the would-be student of these fascinating yet frustrating patients would be puzzled about the entity before him. Was this a real "disease of the mind," marked—like schizophrenia and mania—by no apparent brain pathology and yet revealed by characteristic external symptoms and signs? Was this a thoroughgoing sham, an act of conscious charlatanry or, at least, willful malingering, that counterfeited disease by means of a highly realistic form of drama? Or, more subtly, was this a drama in which the actor had lost control of the role, as it were, and was half agent, half victim of the chosen scenario?

A century later a case report contains these remarks, referring to a middle-aged man who had up to 50 apparently volitional seizures a day (for which he was receiving both medication and disability compensation) and who rapidly stopped seizing when told he could not have solid food if his seizures persisted:

> The question of conversion reaction versus a conscious process is relevant in this case, but the two etiologies have much in common. The difference is largely one of the relative degree to which consciousness participates in the reaction ... conscious and unconscious factors are interwoven in malingering (Poulose and Shaw, 1977).

A century later, then, questions similar to those asked by Charcot's students, questions essentially unresolved, remain to plague the contemporary student of the legal/forensic aspects of nonepileptic seizures.

Before embarking on our discussion, let us acknowledge one caveat. In actual legal practice, a judge and/or jury may decide on a quite idiosyncratic basis to render a particular verdict in a case involving nonepileptic seizures. This matter will be further explored.

For our purposes, let us attempt to differentiate and clarify the legal issues on theoretical grounds by considering six hypothetical cases:

1. A person, driving a car while actively hallucinating that he is actually driving a collision car at an amusement park, hits a pedestrian.
2. A person, driving a car while intoxicated, hits a pedestrian.
3. A person, driving a car, falls asleep and hits a pedestrian.
4. A person, driving a car, sees a pedestrian stranger crossing the road who resembles a hated rival; momentarily *paralyzed* by emotional conflict, the driver hits the pedestrian.
5. A person, driving a car and succumbing to an epileptic seizure, hits a pedestrian.
6. A person, driving a car, succumbs to a psychogenic seizure and hits a pedestrian. (Although pseudoseizures usually occur in circumstances that render injury a rare event, the reader is asked to suspend disbelief for didactic reasons in these examples.)

The clinicolegal questions might then be posed: Is the sixth case of altered "normal" consciousness similar to and/or different from any or all of the other five, and on what grounds? The answer to this question will largely determine how the nonepileptic seizures are considered in relation to criminal responsibility and to competency and how questions of liability (in patients or treaters) are answered.

CRIMINAL RESPONSIBILITY

> When Prince Mishkin, in an epileptic seizure, flails his arms and breaks a valuable vase, it is not too implausible here to say that his body moved without a desire that it move or without any volition that it move (Murphy, 1971).

The question of criminal responsibility is addressed in most jurisdictions by the American Law Institute (ALI) standard which holds a person not responsible if "as a result of mental illness or defect he lacks substantial capacity either to appreciate the criminality of his conduct or to conform his conduct to the requirements of the law" (American Law Institute Model Penal Code, 1962). Although providing some guidance to the clinician, expert-witness, or trier-of-fact, this is a rather vague test.

Using our examples against this principle we realize that it was largely constructed to apply to the first instance: the psychotic whose clear mental illness wreaks havoc with his perceptions of an action in the situation and thus with his capacities to "appreciate" and to "conform" as stated. Intoxication and sleep (in the next examples), although representing impairments, are not considered "mental illnesses" or defect and are thus not covered by the rule. However, drunk driving (itself a crime) or sleep may be entered as a plea of mitigating circumstance. Thus, "accident" might be the ruling rather than "negligence."

The next two cases, the emotionally paralyzed driver and the "true" epileptic, are more instructive, especially in relation to the case of nonepileptic seizures. In the former instance, the driver's paralysis could be said to result from *unconscious conflict*. The dynamic formulation of the incident might delineate how the wishes to harm the rival—wishes operative even though not brought to awareness—vie with humane constraints against harm to others, producing the stalemate expressed in motor *paralysis*; likewise, the origin of the motor *activity* of an hysterical seizure could also be traced to unconscious conflict intolerable to conscious awareness.

"True" epilepsy might be entered as a "defect" in the ALI standard, since that term is usually understood to refer to neurological entities (e.g., retardation) rather than psychological ones. A jury would probably treat it as a biologic accident such as falling asleep at the wheel; mere sleepiness is not excusable, but narcolepsy might well be. Still, the question might be raised: Should a person susceptible to seizures, like a person intoxicated, prevent himself or be prevented from driving? In this regard, a number of states require people with epilepsy to receive medical clearance to be granted a driver's license, often with certain stipulations (e.g., no seizures on medication for 1 year). This question is further explored later in the chapter. Note also Gunn and Fenton (1971) on epileptic automatism as a legal defense (American Law Institute Model Penal Code, 1962).

In Great Britain, interestingly, the Royal Commission on Capital Punishment, weighing different forms of epilepsy as they might relate to homicide, concluded that, in violence occurring in states of postepileptic automatism and "epileptic insanity," " . . . the accused would be wholly irresponsible for this act" (Macrae, 1969). Macrae also probes the difficulties for the judicial process in needing to assess, first, the question of diminished responsibility for epileptic criminals (often expressed as a reduced charge, e.g., homicide reduced to manslaughter) and, second, whether long prison terms, shortened prison terms or indefinite state hospital commitment represented the appropriate dispositions of such cases (Macrae, 1969).

In Australia, Stevenson (1963) described a petty theft case in which the defense of epileptic automatism was accepted by a court; the patient had a clear epileptogenic focus on EEG, good moral character and record and a history of postconcussive "episodes" that were abolished posttrial by anticonvulsant medication. The author notes that this case appeared valid in contrast to the number of specious claims for this entity.

For the hysterical "epileptic" patient, however, these questions are much murkier. Like all the examples *except* the emotionally paralyzed driver, the hysterical seizure victim is in an altered state of consciousness or awareness; like all the examples without exception, the patient's motility is affected; like the sleeping and the paralyzed drivers, and unlike the others, the patient could throw off the altered state of consciousness in reaction to some inner or outer stimulus (waking up, breaking the paralysis by effort of will); and, like all but the sleeper and the epileptic, the hysteric usually is believed to maintain *some* awareness of the surroundings (hence, the rarity of self-injury). On another level, some precautionary actions (getting enough sleep, abstention from alcohol, etc.) might have prevented the injury in some of the examples and, of course, refraining from driving would have served as a universal preventive. One might at this point compare hysterical seizures to two other entities that often present as altered states of consciousness and motility without electroencephalographic findings: sleepwalking and episodic dyscontrol syndrome.

Sleepwalking is usually treated as a nonpsychotic disorder that confers nonresponsibility on the person who commits crimes during one of these episodes; the disorder is considered to interfere with both perceptual awareness and choice of action (Morse, 1967).

The matter of the episodic dyscontrol syndrome (EDS) is far more complex. While somnambulism is a phenomenon recognized not only by physicians but also by laymen for centuries (e.g., Lady Macbeth), EDS is not only a newly defined entity (the past 20 years) but also one with complicating associations to political interpretation of brain or behavioral phenomena. Ratner and Shapiro (1979), for example, describe how intensive neuropsychiatric evaluation led to testimony that partially exonerated a murderer from criminal responsibility, an outcome based on the alleged presence of EDS. The authors note that the clinical value of care in making this diagnosis is the hope that the disorder is remediable through anticonvulsant medication. Other authors find the correlations far more cloudy and uncertain; Hill and Pond (1952), in their review of 100 capital cases in England in which the defendants were examined by EEG, comment on the use of epileptiform automatism as a defense in hopeless cases—a defense that is rarely accepted by the court. A number of authors also point to the complicating role of alcohol in both EDS and epilepsy, sometimes acting through pathologic intoxication (Ratner and Shapiro, 1979; Hill and Pond, 1952; Marinacci and Von Hagen, 1972).

At this time, it appears that EDS has not been defined as a forensic entity with sufficient clarity to permit generalizations about the outcome of such cases. Further, since EDS has not been made an official DSM-III diagnosis, it would be anticipated that pleading its presence would be more difficult than raising defenses based upon more conventional diagnostic entities (American Psychiatric Association, 1979).

THE PROBLEM FOR THE COURT

To grasp the conceptual problem facing the court, it is useful to conceptualize the two extreme forms of these seizures: the pure hysterical (i.e., unconsciously motivated) seizure and the pure malingering (i.e., consciously motivated) seizure. Legally speaking, dealing with malingering is straightforward. Since it is a volitional act, and therefore presumptively under control of the person involved, it would not fall under the ALI test of insanity. That is, a person who was choosing to behave so as to simulate a conventional disease, in this case epilepsy, would still appreciate the criminality of his conduct and be able to conform that conduct to the requirements of law. Thus, malingered seizures present little conceptual difficulty (although the unsophisticated court may be capable of blurring the distinction here being made).

The matter of hysterical seizures, however, is more difficult for the courts and for inexperienced clinicians to conceptualize, in part because nonepileptic seizures (hysterical or malingered) generally occur in those individuals who have epileptic seizures as well. Thus, in most kinds of litigation, in which the presence of seizures was raised to bar liability or criminal responsibility, the defense would probably attempt to demonstrate that a "real" seizure had taken place. For instructional purposes, it is still useful to imagine pure-culture hysterical seizures and a legal defense based upon them.

In order to understand how the law would treat such a defense, one needs to know how the law has traditionally dealt with the hysterical dissociation and hysterical conversion reactions. In the main, these conditions have not served as an adequate basis for an ALI insanity defense. The reason for this is complex. On the face of it, it would appear that somebody who is in a dissociated state (e.g., a hysterical fugue) would be like the somnambulist discussed above, incapable of appreciating the criminality of his/her conduct and of conforming that conduct to the requirements of the law. However, the courts have balked at applying this reasoning to hysterical symptoms, apparently believing as a matter of policy that such an application would open a

"Pandora's box" of spurious and difficult-to-evaluate legal defenses and would make a shambles of the traditional insanity tests which tend to focus on psychosis. Clinically, there is a sound rationale for the court's reticence in this regard: neurotic conditions, and *a fortiori* hysterical ones, are believed to involve some measure of conscious (as well as unconscious) volitional control as suggested earlier. These conditions usually do not produce the kind of sweeping and profound rent in the reality-testing mechanism which is the hallmark of psychosis. Still, no hard-and-fast rule can be articulated about the receptivity of the courts to hysterical seizures as a defense. This has several reasons: the law's continual evolution or the presence of special circumstances may make a particular case especially worthy of excuse (and thus a defense based on a hysterical condition may be allowed even though it does not fit the formal requirements of the law); adroit advocacy, moreover, may sometimes persuade a jury (or judge) to employ a previously untested legal rubric.

Are the limits of criminal responsibility different among healthy people, people with epilepsy, people with hysterical seizures, and people with other causes of episodic alterations of consciousness (e.g., hypoglycemia, cardiac arrhythmia, porphyria or pheochromocytoma)? As outlined above, the answer is yes; *clinical responsibility varies with each of these groups.* This follows from the general rule that people are held legally responsible (either criminally or civilly) for the natural consequences of their acts and from the general exception: unless *those acts* are a *manifestation of a disease.* In the main, then, a person who suffers from a syncopal episode and causes an accident would not be held responsible if the condition had previously not occurred.

To summarize, then, we would say the following: the presence of hysterical seizures raises the possibility of an insanity defense, but historically such defenses have not been allowed, and although this might change in the future, success of this defense would appear unlikely unless there were other factors which would strongly move the court in the direction of mitigation. This stands in contrast to malingering, where there would be essentially no possibility of legitimately raising an insanity defense. Other nonepileptic phenomena would be exculpatory only insofar as the court in question accepted the fact that veritable disease was probably present.

THE QUESTION OF COMPETENCE IN NONEPILEPTIC SEIZURES

The theoretical basis for competence to stand trial and competence to perform certain functions is briefly reviewed in general terms at this point; competence to sign a contract and make a will are reviewed later in this text.

The person with nonepileptic seizures exists in two states of competence in the eyes of the law: the interictal state (between seizures) during which the person is presumably competent, in the absence of compelling evidence to the contrary, and the ictal state (during the seizure) in which the person is probably incompetent.

In this regard, the pattern of competence resembles that of true epilepsy; this resemblance may include the presence of implied consent during a seizure: this means that a person in the ictal state may have treatment administered to him/her without formal consent (Mills et al., 1980). The reasoning here is that the degree of disturbance is so profound, and the impairment of competence is so clear, that consent may be implied as is the case with the comatose patient.

PRACTICAL CONSIDERATIONS

The practicing clinician should be aware of certain practical considerations deriving from the information presented above. An important question is: What is the responsibility (if any) of the treating physician for acts committed by a person having hysterical seizures? As a general rule there is no legal responsibility (liability) on the part of the physician for the acts of his/her patients. The only broadly recognized exception to this doctrine has been those situations in which psychiatrists knew or should have known that their patient was homicidal or otherwise represented a danger to others (Tarasoff v. Regents of the University of California, 1976). In that context, there still exists an ill-defined duty to protect the intended victim. Still, the law is increasingly recognizing an inchoate duty on the part of physicians to prevent harm to others as a result of a patient's disease. This rule developed originally in relation to communicable diseases, where physicians were historically required to report those cases to public agencies (Jacobsen v. Massachusetts, 1905). At present, clinicians treating patients with seizures or pseudoseizures may well be required to counsel their patients not to put themselves in positions where their condition would be apt to endanger others (e.g., driving automobiles, operating heavy machinery or weapons). That is, physicians should warn patients with *all* seizures, irrespective of etiology, of the importance of safeguarding themselves and others. As is generally the case in clinical matters with legal import, the prudent clinician should also briefly but clearly document that warning in the medical record (Gutheil, 1980; Masland, 1978).

What are the legal ramifications of persons susceptible to pseudoseizures operating automobiles, and are these ramifications different from those that apply to the patient with epilepsy? In the arena of civil litigation, both defendants and attorneys have more leeway than in criminal litigation. Legal defenses do not have to fit the historic requirements of the insanity test (the ALI test) or the diminished-capacity doctrine. For tort (personal injury) litigation, the question often depends on the scope of the risk. For example, if one has a history of epilepsy and drives, is it within the scope of foreseeable risk that one will have a seizure and that—as a result of that seizure—another will be injured? In general, the courts have answered in the affirmative, and thus liability has been imposed. As noted below, if one has had no previous history of seizures and no obvious prodrome, courts have not imposed liability, the theory being that liability is excused in the presence of an ineluctable medical condition. Similarly, if one had a history of hysterical seizures, drove, and injured another as a result, one would anticipate liability. But what of the driver who sustains his/her first hysterical seizure? Again, this is a difficult matter. Undoubtedly, much would turn on the apparent equities involved; that is, what appeared fair to judge and jury. The harder question has to do with the amount of "volitional override potential" available to the patient with such seizures. We would speculate that courts would be loath to excuse liability. Fortunately, such matters are rare; unfortunately, because they *are* so rare, the case-law is not adequate to give conclusive answer. Injuries as a result of a malingered seizure would probably be considered as an intentional, as opposed to a negligent, tort so that tortious liability could be even greater.

What are the limits of responsibility for entering into contracts and making wills when a person has had nonepileptic, episodic alterations of consciousness? Reviewing established legal doctrines regarding contractual or testamentary capacity may be useful. Once a contract has vested—that is, once there is a valid offer and acceptance—in order for one party successfully to defend against the obligations of the contract, that party has to demonstrate a lack of contractual capacity *at the time* the contract was signed. Generally, therefore, most episodic disorders do not affect contractual capacity as earlier implied. If the contracting party was awake and alert enough to read and sign the contract, the contract is presumed binding. Clearly, if the party were in the midst of having an epileptic seizure, a hysterical seizure, or even a factitious seizure, he/she would not be able to sign a contract.

Comparable analysis would lead to the identical result insofar as wills are concerned, but such restatements of the law without regard to the subtleties involved in a particular case may obscure important potential nuances. Consider, for example, the nonepileptic seizure that mimics temporal lobe or petit mal epilepsy rather than the more typical major motor seizure. If it were alleged that those conditions were occurring during the time the contract or will was under consideration, their presence might well allow the terms of the contract or will to be excused. Two important considerations apply: first, it would be very difficult to demonstrate that the hysterical, fugue-like state had been experienced at the exact time the contract or will was being drawn; second, the law would probably consider the contract or will valid because hysterical as well as other neurotic conditions are generally not held to be sufficiently disturbing so as to invalidate formalized obligations, as earlier implied. The courts have described the so-called reliance interest of the parties; this states, in effect, that, since both parties have formally agreed by signing, both have certain reasonable expectations. Only extraordinary and compelling circumstances justify setting aside those expectations. Finally, we believe that "straightforward" malingered seizures would not provide a basis to excuse the duty of a contract or the bequests of a will.

CONCLUSIONS AND RECOMMENDATIONS

1. Although the traditional legal rubric for granting either exculpation or diminished responsibility/liability looks to the presence of major psychologic incapacity (e.g., psychosis or organic state), pseudoseizures *may* represent a significantly altered state of consciousness and thus may well impinge upon legal decision-making.
2. These problems are confounded by the clinical observation that "true" seizures, pseudoseizures and malingered seizures may well occur in the same individual; this clinical reality blurs the precise legal distinctions regarding competence, responsibility and capacity.
3. As is the case with true seizures, the clinician acquires an affirmative *duty to warn the pseudoseizure patient* about possible consequences and harms that may result from this condition and to *document that warning.*
4. Tactically, the prudent attorney will generally base a "seizure defense" on the presence, first, of "true" seizures and will proffer pseudoseizures (with their attendant ambiguities and difficulties of proof) as a fallback position.
5. Finally, it is important to remember that, just as good management of the specific clinical condition requires attention to individual variability, so the legal outcome of a given case will be significantly affected by unpredictable factors outside the clinical sphere; these may include the apparent perceived fairness of the situation, the judge's or jury's interest and clinical sophistication, and the skill of the respective advocates.

References

American Law Institute Model Penal Code, 1962: Proposed Office Draft 4.01.

American Psychiatric Association: *Diagnostic and Statistical Manual of Mental Disorders*, ed. 3. Washington, D.C., 1979.

Charcot, J.M. *Clinical Lectures on Certain Diseases of the Nervous System: Lecture VII*, translated by Hurd, E.P. Davis, Detroit, 1888.

Freud, S. Moral responsibility for the content of dreams. In *Collected Papers V*. 1925, p. 157.

Gunn, J., and Fenton, G. Epilepsy, automatism and crime. *Lancet* i:1173–1176, 1971.

Gutheil, T.G. Paranoia and progress notes: A guide to forensically informed psychiatric record keeping. *Hosp. Community Psychiatry* 31:479–482, 1980.

Havens, L.L. *Approaches to the Mind*. Little, Brown & Co., Boston, 1973.

Hill, D., and Pond, D.A. Reflections on one hundred capital cases submitted to electroencephalography. *J. Ment. Sci.* 98:23–43, 1952.

Jacobsen v. Massachusetts, 197 U.S. 11, 1905.

Macrae, A.K.M. Criminal responsibility and epilepsy. In *Current Problems in Neuro-Psychiatry*. British Journal of Psychiatry Special Publication #4, 1969, chap. 14, pp. 87–89.

Marinacci, A.A., and Von Hagen, K.O. Alcohol and temporal lobe dysfunction. *Behav. Neuropsychiatry* 3:2–11, 1972.

Masland, R. The physician's responsibility for epileptic drivers. *Ann. Neurol.* 4:485–486, 1978.

Mills, M.J., Hsu, L.C., Berger, P.D. Informed consent: Psychotic patients and research. *Bull. Am. Acad. Psychiatry Law* 8:119–132, 1980.

Moore, M.S. Responsibility for unconsciously motivated action. *Int. J. Law Psychiatry* 2:323–347, 1979.

Morse, H.N. The physician and the somnambulist. *J.A.M.A.* 199:289–290, 1967.

Murphy, J.G. Involuntary acts and criminal liability. *Ethics* 81:332–342, 1971.

Poulose, K.P., and Shaw, A.A. Rapidly recurring seizures of psychogenic origin. *Am. J. Psychiatry* 134:1145–1146, 1977.

Ratner, R.A., and Shapiro, D. The episodic dyscontrol syndrome and criminal responsibility. *Bull. Am. Acad. Psychiatry Law* 7:422–431, 1979.

Stevenson, H.G. Psychomotor epilepsy associated with criminal behavior. *Med. J. Aust.* 60:784–785, 1963.

Tarasoff v. Regents of the University of California, 551 P. 2d 334, 131 Cal. Rptr. 14, 1976.

Index